From the Womb
to the Tomb

From the Womb to the Tomb:

Issues in Medical Ethics

Hugh V. McLachlan

Centre for Ethics in Public Policy and Corporate Governance, School of Law and Social Sciences Glasgow Caledonian University

J. Kim Swales

The Fraser of Allander Institute, Department of Economics, University of Strathclyde

humming earth

Published by

Humming Earth
an imprint of
Zeticula
57 St Vincent Crescent
Glasgow
G3 8NQ
Scotland.

http://www.hummingearth.com
admin@hummingearth.com

ISBN-13 978-1-84622-011-1 Paperback
ISBN-10 1 84622 011 4 Paperback

ISBN-13 978-1-84622-10-4 Hardback
ISBN-10 1 84622 010 6 Hardback

Acknowledgements

We would like to thank the editors and publishers of the following publications for permission to reprint previously published material: *Analysis; Contemporary Review*; *Health Care Analysis*; *Human Reproduction and Genetic Ethics*; *International Journal of Sociology and Social Policy; Journal of Medical Ethics*; *The Scotsman*. It is indicated in the text where and when previously published chapters were first published.

Thirty Years Worth of Valued Contributions to Medical Ethics

From the Womb to the Tomb: Issues in Medical Ethics by Hugh McLachlan and Kim Swales constitutes a remarkable intellectual journey spanning some 30 years of academic and journalistic contributions by two Glasgow-based thinkers on matters of medical ethics. The oldest paper in this reader was published in the leading philosophy journal *Analysis* back in 1977. I was 13 years old then and did not even know that medical ethics existed or that my career would eventually lead me to engage in thinking on issues in bioethics in a fulltime capacity some years down the track.

Looking at recent debates in Scotland over anti-smoking legislation, egalitarian access principles in the NHS or stem cell research, it is surprising how up-to-date even articles appear to be that were published by McLachlan and Swales many years ago. Given the embarrassing lack of support for medical ethics research and education in most of Scotland's medical schools it is reassuring that intellectuals such as Hugh McLachlan and Kim Swales continue to contribute to leading professional journals. Equally as important, I should think, are their continuing interventions in public debates in Scotland, be they on smoking, commercial surrogacy or justice and fairness in the NHS.

After all, medical ethics as a sub-discipline of ethics would arguably fail if it didn't engage with issues that are of practical concern. It is good to see that this anthology includes content offered initially for 'public consumption', so to speak, namely a paper published in *The Scotsman* on reproductive human cloning. It is proof that good academic analysis does not always have to be hidden away from public view in academic journals. The authors' decision to reprint many of their best publications in medical ethics in this book is to be applauded.

No doubt, on reading the individual articles the reader will, as I have, find himself or herself sometimes in disagreement, and sometimes in agreement with the authors. Whatever your considered views are, the great value this book will have contributed is that it challenged you to reflect on refreshingly original thinking on a wide range of issues of public policy importance. Sometimes it is necessary to be provoked by disagreement with others to develop one's own views more clearly. Indeed, some of the proponents of positions criticized by McLachlan and Swales have done so. St.-Andrews-based Roman Catholic philosopher John Haldane and Oxford-based secular bioethicist Julian Savulescu are just two such colleagues.

I have no doubt that reading this anthology will stimulate the reader's thinking about vitally important issues in health care. It certainly has made me rethink some of the issues under consideration in the pages that follow.

Udo Schuklenk
Co-Editor BIOETHICS

Contents

Abortion

Chapter One

Must We Accept Either the Conservative or the Liberal View on Abortion?*

I

When considering the morality of abortion, it has been common to focus attention upon the ontological status of the fetus and, specifically, to ask whether or not the fetus is a person. Indeed, as Hare points out, the question of:

'. . . whether the fetus is a person, has been so universally popular that in many of the writings it is assumed that this question is the key to the whole problem. The reason for this is easy to see; if there is a well-established moral principle that the intentional killing of other innocent persons is always murder, and therefore wrong, it looks as if an easy way to determine whether it is wrong to kill fetuses is to determine whether they are persons, and thus settle once for all whether they are subsumable under the principle (R. M. Hare, 'Abortion and the Golden Rule', *Philosophy and Public Affairs*, vol. 4, 1975, p. 204).

If we approach the abortion issue in this way, then it appears that abortion is never, or almost never, justifiable or else never in need of justification:

'For, if a human fetus is a person, one is inclined to say that, in general, one would be justified in killing it only to save the life of the mother. Such is the extreme conservative position. On the other hand, if the fetus is not a person, how can it be seriously wrong to destroy it?' (M. Tooley, 'Abortion and Infanticide', *Philosophy and Public Affairs*, vol. 2, 1972, pp. 38-39).

That it is never wrong to destroy it is the extreme liberal position. There appears to be no plausible middle ground between the extreme conservative and the extreme liberal views on abortion. I want to argue that this appearance is deceptive and that the deception is produced by a misrepresentation of the ontological status of the fetus and of the importance of this status.

What is the ontological status of the fetus ? According to Hare, this is a moral question. For reasons that need not concern us here, he thinks that ' ... to say that the fetus becomes a person at conception, or at quickening, or at birth, or whenever takes your fancy ... is inescapably a moral decision for which we have to have moral reasons' (Hare, p. 205). An opposing point of view is presented by, for example, Werner. He distinguishes a 'human being' by which term he means '... a member of the biological species *homo sapiens*' from a 'person' which is said to be ' . . . a fully fledged member of a human community, someone having a developed concept of self, memories, a language and/or moral obligations as well as moral rights . . .' (R. Werner, 'Hare on Abortion', *Analysis* 36.4, 1976, p. 178). He concludes that fetuses are not persons but are human beings: they are '. . . the live, growing uterine offspring of human beings and are not members of any other plant or animal species' (Werner, p. 179). Both writers have committed a simple category error which commonly occurs in the abortion debate. Is the fetus a person or is it a human being? When does the fetus become a person or a human being? A fetus is neither a person nor a human being; a fetus never becomes a person or a human being: it is or might become the body of one. In at least one respect, the question of the ontological status of the fetus is quite unproblematical and non-moral. A fetus is a partially developed human body (I argue this in 'Moral Rights and Abortion', *Contemporary Review*, vol. 228, no. 1325, June 1976, pp. 323-8).

People sometimes ask what, if any, are the rights of the fetus and this is a curious question. We never attribute rights to fully developed bodies so why should we attribute them to partially developed ones ? After all, we would not say that my arms or legs or any other part of my body, or, indeed, my entire body had rights. It is, rather, me who has rights. Rights are held by people, not by their bodies. Should we therefore conclude that the extreme liberal position is firmly established and that since a fetus cannot have rights, abortions are not in need of justification when the prospective mothers desire them? We can validly reach this conclusion only by making two assumptions which can be challenged. Consider Tooley's claim that: 'Settling the issue of the morality of abortion and infanticide will involve answering the following questions: What properties must something have to be a person, i.e. to have a serious right to life ? At what point in the development of a member of the species *homo sapiens* does the organism possess the properties that make it a person?' (Tooley, p. 43). The assumptions to which I refer are being made here by Tooley. Firstly, it is assumed not only that rights are due only to persons but that such persons must be living, actual persons. Secondly, it is assumed that in order for us to have duties regarding abortion, there must be someone possessing corresponding rights.

Let us deal with these assumptions in turn. Suppose we promise a friend that we shall never reveal a particular secret. Are we released from our duty not to break our trust on our friend's death? Can we not say that he still has a right not to have his confidence betrayed and that we have a duty not to betray it? Suppose we promise to place flowers on his grave. It seems to me that our dead friend has a right to have flowers placed on his grave and that we have a corresponding duty to place them there. And such duties to the dead need not arise through contract or personal relationships. I never met Wittgenstein. Yet, I would suggest that I have duties towards the dead man. For example, I have a duty not to slander him and it is not an obvious abuse of language to say that he has a right not to be slandered. To say the least, it is not self-evident that only actual living persons have rights. We might say that the person whose body a fetus might develop into has rights and that, correspondingly, we have duties towards him whether or not he is an actual living person or ever will become one. We can have duties towards the person who might or will become the occupier of a particular body if a fetus develops into a fully formed human body. If I am correct in maintaining that a non-existent person can have rights and that we can have duties towards him, then the question of the ontological status of the fetus need not be considered to be critically important and certainly not the central issue in the abortion debate. We need not be particularly concerned with the question whether the fetus is the partially formed body of an actual person or of a human being or the question at what precise stage a fetus, or, indeed, the body of a baby becomes that of an actual person or human being.

We might even talk of our having duties towards persons whose bodies are not yet fetuses. Suppose someone knew that if he were to have sex with his wife at a particular time then the human being who would be produced would live in abject misery because of, say, some physical ailment. He would surely have a duty not to have sex at that particular time and why should we shy from saying that the miserable person who would be produced has a right against him that he does not have sex at that particular time? If talk of rights with non-existent holders seems peculiar then it could be said simply that he has a duty not to have sex at that particular time and that no one holds a corresponding right. This leads us to the second assumption to be considered.

It is doubtful whether on every occasion when we have a duty to do X, in the sense that we ought to do X, that X be done is some particular person's right. Suppose that we were living in a country where many people around us were starving and that we had far more food than we needed for both our present and our future purposes. We would surely have a duty to give some of our food away, in the sense that we ought to do so, even if it were the case that no particular person had a right to receive food from us. We might have enough spare food to feed only one person and have a duty to feed one starving person where no starving person had any more right to receive the food than had any other. Consider our conservation policies or our moral concern at their relative absence. Suppose that all the world's natural resources will run out in one hundred years if we continue with our present rate of consumption and that the earth, and all other planets, will be unfit for human habitation. Should we be morally concerned at this possible state? Would we not think it immoral for us avoidably to act in such a way that future human life would be precluded? Even if we were to deny that the members of potential generations have rights, I am sure that most of us would assert that we have a duty not to dissipate natural resources just as we would have a duty not to waste food in the company of starving people even if no one is the holder of a corresponding right. Once again, if we can have moral duties without there being holders of corresponding rights, then the question of the ontological status of the fetus and of whether this status is such that the fetus could reasonably be considered to be the holder of rights need not be considered central or critical in determining the morality of abortion.

II

Before considering an alternative to the extreme liberal and extreme conservative views on abortion, I want to discuss some further arguments for the liberal view.

It might be thought that if the fetus is simply a partially formed human body then it is the property of the woman who carries it and that she is morally entitled to do what she wants with it. It might be thought that abortion is no more a moral issue than tooth extraction. Is it not the case, as Thomson claims, that '. . . the mother and the unborn child are not like two tenants in a small house which has, by an unfortunate mistake, been rented to both: the mother owns the house'? (J. J. Thomson, 'A Defense of Abortion', *Philosophy and Public Affairs*, vol. 2, 1972, p. 5 3). It is curious to talk of ownership in relation to any bodies, most of all fetuses. For instance, when we own a house we can sell it and cease to own it, but, even if we were prostitutes or slaves, our bodies would, indeed must, in an obvious sense remain our own. Is Thomson talking about legal ownership or what we might call 'logical ownership'; or is some notion of 'moral ownership' involved? If the fetus is that of the mother, is it not also that of the father? Furthermore, could the fetus not be thought to 'belong' to the person into whose body it might develop? It is his body after all. It is not clear who, if anyone, is the sole 'owner' of the fetus and it is not clear in what sense, if any, it is appropriate to talk of ownership in relation to the fetus.

Nevertheless, it might be thought that the fetus is part of a woman's body. What would follow from this? Is a woman entitled to do with it as she pleases because of her '. . . right to decide what happens in and to her body which everyone seems ready to grant'? (Thomson, p. 50). It is not clear that anyone has such a right. A right to decide what happens to one's body might be the absence of duties towards other people to treat our bodies in particular ways. But we are surely not free of such duties. Would a husband not be failing in his duty towards his wife if he took a drug such as heroin to such an extent the he was never capable of sex and failing in his duty towards his children if he abused his body in such a way that it was never capable of work? The fact that a fetus is part of a woman's body does not preclude her having duties regarding its disposal towards the person whose body the fetus might become. To have a right to decide what happens to one's body might mean that there is nothing which one ought to do or ought not to do with one's body; it might mean that there is an absence of all duties regarding its use and not just of duties with corresponding rights. Even if no one had a right to our bodies or a right to a particular performance from them, we might still have duties regarding our bodies. We might have a duty to keep our bodies healthy even if no one has a right that our bodies are healthy. A woman might 'own' a fetus totally in the sense that no one has a right that it is treated in any particular way and yet have duties regarding its disposal just as we would have duties regarding the disposal of our own food in a land of starving people. For example, we might imagine a situation where the birth-rate had declined to such an extent that the human race was in serious danger of extinction. A woman then might have a duty to have a baby rather than an abortion even though no one else had any rights regarding the treatment of her fetus. We might think that it is morally good to perpetuate human life even if we did not think that any particular person had a right to be born. In some other situation, a woman might be morally obliged to have an abortion even if it were no one's right that she had one.

The following objection is raised by Tooley against the view that currently non-existent persons can have rights. He asks us to imagine a situation where:

'... a chemical [is] discovered which when injected into the brain of a kitten would cause the kitten to develop into a cat possessing a brain of the sort possessed by humans and consequently into a cat having all the psychological capabilities characteristic of adult humans. Such cats would be able to think, to use language and so on. Now it would surely be morally indefensible in such a situation to ascribe a serious right to life to members of the species *homo sapiens* without also ascribing it to cats that have undergone such a process of development; there would be no morally significant differences (Tooley, pp. 60-1).

He then assumes that if a kitten had been injected with a such a chemical it could not be morally wrong to prevent the kitten's developing into a cat with the mentioned human-like qualities and concludes:

'But if it is not seriously wrong to destroy an injected kitten which will naturally develop the properties that bestow a right to life, neither can it be seriously wrong to destroy a member of *homo sapiens* which lacks such properties, but will naturally come to have them' (Tooley, p. 61).

According to Tooley, abortions are not in need of justification and the extreme liberal position is established.

One might reject Tooley's conclusion and insist that it would require justification to kill such injected kittens. Tooley argues that 'It is hard to believe that there is much to be said for the . . . moral claim . . . that in a world in which kittens could be transformed into "rational animals" it would be seriously wrong to kill newborn kittens' (Tooley, p. 62). If he finds this moral claim implausible then this is surely a matter concerning his own psychology or moral judgment; the moral claim appears to me to be one which could rationally be held. Might it not, at least in some circumstances, be wrong wantonly to destroy kittens which would not develop into any thing other than normal cats?

Let us take Tooley's illustration to its logical conclusion. Suppose there were a chemical which when injected into the body of, say, a kitten would cause the body to become that of a person who was like other human persons in every respect other than genealogy.

Suppose that a kitten had just been injected with the chemical. Tooley would claim that this kitten is on a moral par with a normal fetus. Well, we can concede this claim and say that the same moral consideration would be due to the person whose body that of the kitten would become as to any other person whose body developed in the more normal way. It might be that no moral consideration was yet due to any such persons and anyone who claimed that abortion or the killing of the imagined kitten are never in need of any moral justification would be committed to that view. Nevertheless, we are not logically bound to accept the view. We can rationally claim that moral respect and consideration are due to such persons even if we do not want to claim that in all or in any cases they have anything approaching a right to be born.

To the claim that non-existent people can have rights, it might be objected that since they cannot be identified, we cannot have duties towards them and consequently they cannot have rights. Hare considers such an objection and suggests that 'identify' is an ambiguous term. 'I can identify the next man to occupy my carrel at the library by describing him thus, but in another sense I cannot identify him because I have no idea who he is' (Hare, p. 220). He thinks that we can identify the supposed object of the duty to abort or not abort in the former although not in the latter sense: '. . . he is identifiable in the sense that reference can be made to him' (Hare, p. 220). For example, 'The person who will be born if these two people start their coitus in precisely five minutes is identified by that description' (Hare, p. 220). Similarly, as I have done, we can talk of the person whose body a fetus might, will or would have become and that is to identify him. In any case, why should identification be thought important? Well, if I have a duty to give someone a sum of money then it would seem that the person would have to be identifiable in the sense that he could be recognized as the holder of the right, picked out from a crowd as it were, since he would have to be (directly or indirectly) contacted by me in order for me to give him the money. If I could not contact him and know that I had contacted him and not someone else, then it could be argued that it would be impossible for me to fulfil my duty to give him the money and consequently that I do not have a duty to give him the money and he does not have a right against me to its receipt. But the situation is quite different in the case of our duties towards the unborn since it is possible for us to fulfil them without being able to recognize or contact the people involved. We might fulfil our obligations towards the members of future generations by failing to destroy the world without knowing who such people are.

III

We need adopt neither the extreme liberal nor the extreme conservative position on abortion. We can hold that the fetus is neither a person nor a human being nor the body of an actual living person or living human being without being committed to the view that abortions are never in need of a justification. We can assume that it is not only actual living persons who have moral rights and/or that there can be moral duties which do not correspond to a person's rights. We might say that in some, although not necessarily all, cases there is either a duty to abort or a duty not to abort where this duty corresponds to a non-existent person's right and/or we might say that there is simply either a duty to abort or a duty not to abort. Although I have not refuted either the extreme liberal or the extreme conservative positions and have not sought to do so, I have tried to show some of the assumptions behind the positions and that they can be denied. Yet, an extreme liberal might still maintain that when a woman seeks an abortion, such abortion is not in need of a moral justification. He might say that although it is logically possible that non-existent persons have rights, they do not have them in fact; and that although it is logically possible that we have duties on other grounds either to promote or not to promote abortions, as it so happens we do not. He might say that even if non-existent persons have rights, their rights are so weak that we are always justified in not upholding them if they conflict with a potential mother's wishes; and similarly that any other duties which there are pertaining to abortion are comparatively so trivial that a woman's wish to have an abortion will always justify her having one. Similarly, an extreme conservative might maintain that, even though a fetus is not a person nor even the body of an actual living person, abortions are (almost) never justifiable either because of the strength of the rights of the non-existent persons involved or on some other grounds.

What position should we adopt in the abortion issue? I have not tried to answer that question and, apparently unlike some participants in the abortion debate, I consider this to be a straightforward moral question rather than a philosophical one. Between the various possible answers to this moral question, my comments are, I think, ethically neutral. Moral philosophy can indicate the range of possible answers to the question and what assumptions underlie them; moral judgment is required to decide what answers and assumptions are acceptable.

*By Hugh V. McLachlan, from *Analysis*, 1977, vol. 37, no. 4, pp. 197 – 204.

Chapter Two

Bodies, Rights and Abortion*

Abstract

The issue of abortion is discussed with reference to the claim that people have a right of control over their own bodies. Do people "own" their own bodies? If so, what would be entailed? These questions are discussed in commonsense terms and also in relation to the jurisprudence of Hohfeld, Honore, Munzer and Waldron.

It is argued that whether or not women are morally and/or should be legally entitled to have abortions, such entitlements cannot be derived from a general moral entitlement to do what we will with our own bodies since there is no such entitlement. Whether or not we "own " them, we can have rights duties, liabilities, restrictions and disadvantages as well as rights concerning our own bodies.

Introduction

It is sometimes argued, or even implied as a self-evident truth that the pro-abortionists' case rests securely on the assumption that a woman has a fundamental right to do what she will with her own body. I shall question this approach to the abortion debate.

Bodies, rights and common sense

Consider the assumption at issue in the abstract: "That particular X is your X and, therefore, you are entitled to do what you want with it". As a matter of pure logic, the claim is an absurdity. What if "X" stands for a Thompson Machine Gun? Should we say: "That is your machine gun and, therefore, you can do whatever you like with it?" On the contrary, although there might be some things which you and only you can of right do to and with the gun, if that particular machine gun is your machine gun then it is incumbent upon you in particular to ensure that certain things are *not* done with it. Is the situation any different when "X" pertains to one's body or to parts of it? I do not think so. What about: "That is your voice and, therefore, you are entitled to say whatever you like with it"? Certainly not. Concerning what is said with one's own voice, one bears particular obligations of often, for instance, intended reasonableness and truthfulness which one does not bear concerning what other voices say.

Homeowners are morally and legally entitled to paint the

outsides of their front doors any colour they choose. Nonetheless, the entitlement does not derive from an entitlement to do anything they like with their own houses, from a freedom from all obligations concerning how their houses are treated and controlled. Concerning his or her own home, a homeowner has particular *duties* as well as particular rights which other people do not have concerning his or her home. Analogously, we have particular moral duties as well as particular moral rights towards and concerning our own bodies.

According to Shaver:

"The assertion that a woman has the right to control her own body is an unambiguous statement of her proprietorship in her person, and the 'right to choose' an expression of her free will. These claims assume an essential individualism in which the woman properly acts in the pursuit of her own needs and wishes. Her rightful action is limited only by the freedom of others to do likewise".[1]

Consider this together with another of Shaver's claims that:

"The notion of individual rights is quintessentially liberal. At the heart of liberalism lies the proposition that the individual is the rightful possessor of his or her bodily capacities, what MacPherson has termed the ideology of possessive individualism".[2]

Here, Shaver paints only half of the picture of liberalism. It seems strange to talk of "rightful possession" of one's body or of its capacities but, insofar as one might/does, one should say that "rightful possession" of one's body and its capacities is the source of duties no less than of rights concerning it and them. Quintessential to liberalism is the notion of *individual moral autonomy* from which follows equally the potential for the possession of obligations and of rights concerning one's own body.

To say that we have duties concerning our own bodies would seem precisely to place limits on our rights concerning them. These limits are not where Shaver places them. For instance, in the middle of a restaurant, I have, because of my particular duties concerning my body (which I do not have concerning the bodies of other people and they do not have concerning mine) a duty to try not to vomit nor to belch loudly. Nonetheless, *pace* Shaver, my rightful action here is not limited by the rights of others – since in that context they have no such rights – to belch loudly or to vomit.

Again, one might say that most duties which I have, including those physical, emotional and financial ones towards and concerning my wife, can be fulfilled only if my body remains relatively healthy.

I have acquired too, along with our joint mortgage and the related endowment insurance policy, a duty not to commit suicide – an action which would render the policy null and void. One might paraphrase Shaver and say that: the assertion that a person has the *duty* to control his or her own body is an unambiguous statement of "his or her proprietorship in his or her own person" and the *duty* to choose to act in particular ways is an expression of his or her free will. Perhaps this expresses merely a partial truth and perhaps this statement would require qualification to be completely acceptable. Yet, it is no less acceptable as it stands than is Shaver's claim that: "The assertion that a woman has the right to control her own body is an unambiguous statement of her proprietorship in her person, and the 'right to choose' an expression of her free will".[3]

Shaver says that her assertion about rights is "unambiguous". Is it? There are at least two everyday senses in which we talk about rights: rights of action and rights of recipience.

I have a right of action, say, to stand on my head or to pick up a discarded cigar butt from the gutter if and insofar as I am not under any obligation not to stand on my head or to refrain from picking up the cigar butt. If I have such a right to stand on my head or to pick up the cigar butt, then my possession of these rights does not in itself correspond to nor impose obligations on other people. From my possession of these particular rights, other people are not thereby obliged, for instance, to try to help me to stand on my head or to try to help me to pick up the cigar butt. Indeed, someone else in the street, approaching the cigar butt from a different direction from mine might, no less than I have, have a right of action to pick up the cigar butt and pick it up, thereby depriving me of the cigar butt without thereby depriving me of a right.

I have a right of recipience, say, to receive £5 from my next door neighbour and a right of (negative) recipience not to be killed by her if and insofar as she has a duty not to kill me and a duty to give me £5 (which, let us say, she borrowed from me last week). Rights of action are the absences of obligations. Rights of recipience of a person are rights which correspond to the duties of another or of others.

When Shaver says that: "The assertion that a woman has the right to control her own body is an unambiguous statement of her proprietorship in her person . . .", what she is saying is wrong: her assertion *is* ambiguous. She might be talking about a right of action or a right of recipience or both, perhaps, or neither.

The most obvious interpretation, it seems to me, is that she is talking about a moral right of action: the absence of moral obligation. Yet, she might be talking about a moral right of recipience. She might be saying, for instance, that other people have a moral duty not to try to prevent a woman from doing to and with her own body what she will. (She might even mean that other people have a moral duty to try to help a woman to do what she chooses to do to and with her own body.)

In neither sense of the term "right" is it plausible to say *tout court* that, because one's body is one's own, one has a right to do what one wants with it: that one has no moral obligations concerning it; or that others are duty-bound not to interfere with – nor with one's own decisions concerning – one's own body.

Suppose that I stop to pick up a cigar butt or to stand on my head in the middle of a busy road. Other people are not necessarily duty-bound to tolerate my decision to control my body in this way. They might well be entitled – they might even have a duty – forcibly to relocate my body in a more suitable place. Even if I might sometimes have a right of action to stand on my head and to pick up a cigar butt, it does not follow – because my body is mine nor on any other grounds – that at all times and places I have these rights. That X is your X – that hand-grenade is your hand-grenade – yet it does not follow that you have no moral obligations which limit your legitimate use of it. It does not follow that, in any sense of the term, you must have a right to do with it what you will. If "X" stands for one's body or for its capacities, then the logic of the assertion remains the same.

Because, say, one's fertility is a capacity of one's own body, one might have particular rights (perhaps of action and of recipience) concerning it but one will not necessarily be free of all obligations in relation to it nor will all other people thereby necessarily be encumbered with a duty not to interfere with one in one's chosen manner of regulating one's own fertility. They will not necessarily be encumbered with a duty to try to help one to do what one will concerning one's fertility. Concerning one's own fertility, one might have particular duties as well as particular rights of different sorts.

Property, bodies and jurisprudence

According to Munzer:

"In moral philosophy, thinkers have long wrestled with problems of suicide, slavery, self-enslavement, and abortion. Some of the 'solutions' proposed from time to time have either embraced, or repudiated, the idea of owning or having a title to or property rights in oneself as morally relevant. A finer-grained taxonomy, like that advanced here, may help to draw morally pertinent distinctions more clearly than saying, or denying, that persons own their own bodies. The classification of body rights into personal rights and weak and strong property rights may help with these intellectual struggles".[4]

Hohfeld presents a vocabulary of four terms, his inter-related definitions of which he considers to be the basic concepts of law. The terms are: claim-right; privilege; power, and immunity.[5]
A claim-right is what I mean by a right of recipience. As Munzer explains Hohfeld's system of terms:

"A privilege is a legal liberty or freedom. It involves not a correlative duty but the absence of a right on someone else's part to interfere. A claim-right is also quite different from a power. A person has a legal power when, by some act, he can alter his legal position or that of someone else. The correlative of a power is a liability".[6]

For instance, I have a legal power to sell to you -thus altering the legal position of both of us – the word-processor on which I am now working in my home in Paisley. Correlatively, you can have the liability – where a "liability" in Hohfeld's sense need not be disadvantageous – to receive the machine from me. I do not have the legal power to sell to you the computer on which, when I am working at my place of employment, I work although I might have the illegal capacity to do so. Munzer continues:

"Finally, a claim-right differs from an immunity. An immunity is a lack of susceptibility to having one's legal position altered by someone else. . . . If B cannot legally compel A to sell his farm, A has an immunity with respect to B's forcing the sale of the farm. Correlatively, B has no power to force a sale".[6]

Munzer combines Hohfeld's analysis with that of Honore. Munzer says of the latter:

"He sought to specify the standard 'incidents' of ownership common to Western legal systems. These incidents are jointly sufficient, though not individually necessary for ownership. Honore's list of incidents, slightly modified, includes the claim-rights to possess, use, manage, and receive income; the powers to transfer, waive, exclude and abandon; the liberties to consume or destroy; immunities from expropriation; the duty not to use harmfully; and liability for execution to satisfy a court judgment. If a person has all of these incidents, or most of them, with respect to a certain thing, then he or she owns it".[7]

To the question of whether we own our own bodies, Munzer does not give an unqualified "yes" or "no". Because we cannot sell them, he is reluctant to say that we own our own bodies, that they are our property. Munzer argues that, rather than owning our bodies, we have limited property rights in them. Furthermore, he argues, we also have rights other than property rights in and concerning our bodies. An absence of the power of transfer is the defining feature of what Munzer considers to be personal, i.e. non-property body rights. For instance, my right of free speech is, among other things, a right concerning my body since I need to use my voice to speak. However, since I cannot transfer my right of free speech to another person in the sort of way that I can, say, sell my word-processor or my hair, it is not a property right. You might use what used to be my word-processor: you could not use what used to be my right of free speech. You can possess and use more than one word-processor: you cannot similarly possess and use more than one right of free speech. For Munzer, weak as opposed to strong property rights exist when there is the power to transfer but not to sell.

Munzer writes:

"Taken jointly, the body rights of each person amount not to ownership but only a weaker package of limited property rights. Considered individually, the body rights of each person are not all in the same boat. Most body rights are personal rather than property rights; examples are rights not to be murdered, not to be searched without a warrant or just cause, not to be compelled to testify against oneself, not to be libelled or slandered, to speak freely, and to exclude others from sexual or other physical contact. Some body rights are property rights -whether weak such as rights to donate an organ upon death or strong, such as the right of publicity or the right to sell blood or semen; but these weak or strong rights are neither so numerous nor so central as to establish that persons 'own' themselves".[8]

Even if we do not own our bodies, we can still have rights (and duties) concerning them, as Munzer's analysis suggests. Munzer also shows that, as a general thing, property ownership carries duties, liabilities and disadvantages as well as rights. Hence, I think that we can say, even if we do own our bodies, we can still have duties and so forth (and rights) concerning them. Munzer writes:

"The idea *of property rights* is narrower than that of property. Property rights involve only advantageous incidents. Property involves disadvantageous incidents as well. Meant here is advantage or disadvantage to the right-holder or owner. Although property obviously involves disadvantages to persons other than the right-holder, it is important to see that there can be disadvantages to the right-holder as well. Suppose that someone owns a single-family home in a suburban area. Then she has a duty not to use it in ways prohibited by the law of nuisance or by zoning regulations. She may be disabled from transferring it to others with burdensome restrictions – for example, that no one may use it save for unduly limited purposes. If someone wins a court judgment for damages against her, then, subject perhaps to homestead laws, she has a liability that the homestead be sold to pay the judgment. The duty, disability, and liability are disadvantageous to her. It would be odd to say that they are part of her property rights in her home. But they are part of what is involved in saying that the home is her property".[9]

Waldron also emphasises that ownership of property entails liabilities as well as their opposites.[10] However, Waldron is less reluctant than Munzer to deny on the basis of non-transferability that we cannot own our own bodies. He writes:

"I can be the owner of something in the sense that it is for me rather than for anyone else to make decisions about its use (and in the sense that society will back up my decisions with force if need be), without it being the case that I can, by my say-so, transfer exactly that power of decision over the resource to somebody else"."

In discussing Locke's theory of property, Waldron notes that:

"Locke does not say or require in his theory of appropriation that we should have property rights in our bodies. The term he uses is '*person*': 'every man has a Property in his own Person. This no Body has any Right to but himself... given the general character of his position, it is much more plausible for him to say that a man has creator's rights over his person than that he has them over his body".[12]

This distinction highlights another possible ambiguity in Shaver's treatment of abortion. She talks about both a woman's "proprietorship in her person" and of the individual's being "the rightful possessor of his or her bodily capacities". Are there two sorts of ownership which are being suggested here or does "person" in this context mean "body"?

Conclusion

My own view is that talk of ownership of one's person rather than of one's body is absurd. A person cannot be distinguished here from what the person is being said to own. For it to be possible for A to own X, A and X must be, like a person and a person's body, conceptually separable (even if, like husband and wife, they are conceptually relatable).

I do not know what should be said, overall, about the legal, quasi-legal and moral senses in which one might be said to own one's own body. I am tempted to say that if *only one* person *ever could* own such and such then no one *does* own it. I cannot transfer to another the ability to control my actions *in the way that I am able to control them* and, thus, can be responsible for them. I feel that this sort of responsibility and control is, thereby, something different from property but perhaps my feeling is whimsical. Perhaps we should say that the relationship between ourselves and our bodies is *like* that of normal ownership in some respects but not in others and leave it at that.

Property is a bundle of particular rights, privileges, duties and powers rather than a general duty and/or right. The question of ownership in relation to anything at all is complex. It is no less complex in relation to bodies, including our own. Concerning my body, I can control it in a way that no one else can. Similarly, I need it in a way which no one else does and experience pain and pleasure regarding it in a way which no one else does. From these considerations, and perhaps other ones, arise particular rights, powers, privileges, responsibilities and duties which I have concerning my body and which other people have concerning theirs. In this, I agree with Shaver although I emphasise the possibility of duties no less than of rights.

Whether or not we "own", in any sense of the term, our own bodies and/or our bodily capacities or our "persons" does not seem to be crucial here. Ownership can be a basis of the possession of rights and duties but it is not a prerequisite for their possession. Whether or not we own our bodies and/or our bodily capacities, we can still have rights and duties concerning them. It is not obvious that the answer to the question of whether or not we have property in either our bodies or in our "persons" can settle the issues: does one have a moral entitlement or any other sort of moral right to have an abortion?; should one have a legal entitlement or any other sort of legal right to have an abortion?

I have not tried to argue against the pro-abortionist case as such but against the claim that it can be established in a straightforward way from the assertion that we have property in our bodies or "persons". Independently of whether or not we have such property, we can have rights and duties concerning our own bodies. What these rights and duties happen to be is a question which my comments here leave open.

*By Hugh V. McLachlan from the *Journal of Medical Ethics*, 1997, Vol. 23, No. 3, pp. 176-180. Reproduced with permission from the BMJ publishing group.

References

1 Shaver S. Body rights, social rights and the liberal welfare state. *Critical Social Policy* 1993/1994; 39: 70.
2 See reference 1: 69.
3 See reference 1: 70.
4 Munzer SR. *A theory of property.* Cambridge: Cambridge University Press, 1990:54-5.
5 Hohfeld WN. *Fundamental legal conceptions as applied to judicial reasoning.* Westport: Greenwood Press, 1978.
6 See reference 4: 18.
7 See reference 4: 22-3
8 See reference 4: 57.
9 See reference 4:11
10 Waldron J. *The right to private property.* Oxford: Clarendon Press, 1988:27.
11 See reference 10:399
12 See reference 10: 178-180.

Embryology and Human Cloning

Chapter Three

Harris on Quintavalle and the Ethics of Stem-cell Research*

Prof. John Harris, from Manchester University, has recently given a crude and unfair account of a pro-life position on the ethics and appropriate legal status of stem-cell research [1]. My own views, which are usually in agreement with those of Harris, are normally very far from those of Josephine Quintavalle, whom he cites and satirises. Indeed, I do not think that research on human embryos is unethical. Whether or not it is unethical, I do not think that it should be illegal [2]. Hence, although I want to counter Harris's attack on the pro-life position, I do not seek to specifically defend the latter. However, there are truths at the basis of the pro-life position that are not peculiar to it. Harris might appear to be denying them and thereby presenting a dubious account of the nature of normal moral and political reasoning. For instance, there are some decisions that we should not take and some actions that we should not perform, even if the consequences are the same as, or even worse than, they would have been had we not so decided and acted. Not all good effects are our business to bring about. Some actions are our duties to perform despite of and whatever their consequences.

Harris talks of people: '... like Josephine Quintavalle of the pro-life group Comment on Reproductive Ethics, who believe that "no human life should be sacrificed for the benefit of anybody else, no matter how dramatic the promises are"' adding that:

'Such a view seems to take the moral high ground and to reject any trade-off between lives. But, so far from rejecting a trade off between lives, the pro-life position actually advocates such a trade-off. It says that in a choice between the lives of embryos and the lives of those whom embryo research might save, it is the embryonic lives that must be protected.' [3]

Harris adds in what seems to me(but might not be) a sarcastic tone: 'The ethics of this way of choosing between lives certainly require more attention'. [3]

However, this puts the matter wrongly and unfairly. The 'choice' that Quintavalle makes and advocates might or might not have the outcome that Harris suggests. However, it does not follow that her 'choice' is tantamount to a choice between these outcomes. Our chosen courses of action will, of course, have effects but we should not choose between possible courses of actions on the sole basis of these effects far less on the basis of them indiscriminately. For instance, if I give a particular student 30% for a particular essay, there will be a series of predictable and unpredictable effects that will ensue. If I give instead, 70%, the effects will be different. However, it would be quite wrong of me to allow a consideration of these effects to determine my decision and action. What is morally permissible? What is morally obligatory? In what capacity are we deciding and acting? Such questions need to be addressed and answered. [4]

Suppose that I were in a situation where I had to choose between actions that would lead to the saving of my wife's life or the saving of the life of a foreign stranger. I would and should choose to save the life of my wife because my duties towards her are stronger and deeper than those I have towards the stranger. The relative importance and moral worth of their lives would not be a question at issue. I would not be making nor advocating a moral trade-off between lives. My decision and action would involve a trade-off, if you like, between my competing duties, if I have any that compete, in the circumstances. I would not be saying or implying that other people, if they are confronted with the choice, should choose to save my wife's life rather than the life of the foreign stranger.

I do not believe that Quintavalle has ever said what Harris says or suggests that she said, namely: '.... in a choice between the lives of embryos and the lives of those whom embryo research might save, it is the embryonic lives that must be protected'. If she did say it, Harris should have directly quoted her as having said it. Harris might think that what she says implies what Harris says that she said. However, it does not imply it. In any case, there is a difference between saying X and saying something that implies X. If, for instance, someone – call her Nancy – says that Alfred, a particular colleague of hers, who is a bachelor, has a niece who has become friendly with my step-son, what Nancy says implies all sorts of things. For instance, it implies that Alfred is a brother. However, it might be news to Nancy that Alfred is a brother. It would be wrong to say that Nancy said: 'Alfred is a brother'. In addition, it would be wrong to say or to suggest that she said that Alfred is a brother.

Quintavalle does not say what Harris says that she says. She does say – and it is quite a different thing – the following:

'Where stem cells are harvested from the embryo and foetus as opposed to the umbilical cord or placenta of the newborn or the adult, existing life has to be sacrificed. This is a trade-off which

CORE simply cannot accept. We believe we have a duty to protect human subjects from abuse, and this duty must inform all medical ethics. Regardless of potential benefit, we must reject outright any research which results in the deliberate destruction of human life.... We believe that such cures should never depend on the killing of an unborn child.... Even if embryonic and foetal stem cells were to prove safe and effective in forthcoming decades, the fact remains that they can only be harvested at the cost of destroying early human life. Such cures can never be morally acceptable'.[5]

What she says, quite clearly, is that we should not make such a choice as Harris says that she makes and/or advocates making. If her recommendations were accepted, then it is not true that the lives of embryos will be protected rather than that of living people who might otherwise have benefited from research on embryos. The embryos on which research might have been carried out would not have existed. In a situation where – contrary to Quintavalle's recommendations – embryos have been created in order that research may be conducted on them, it is her view that the envisaged research should not be carried out. In other words, she would say that on the grounds that no human life should be sacrificed for the sake of another human life, the research should not take place. Whether the life of an embryo is worth more than the life of a mature sick human being is not at stake. Harris is wrong in suggesting that a question that is not being explicitly addressed is being answered implicitly here. It would be better were the question not raised. If it is asked – as an idle fancy in the privacy of our own mind – we should not act upon our answer to it. Quintavalle – not Harris – is right, on this point at least.

For example, suppose that someone thought that abortion should be legal. It would be wrong to say that such a conclusion was an implicit assessment that the life of an embryo or foetus was of less value than that of a pregnant woman, although the explicit assessment that such is so might lead some people to conclude that abortion should be legal. For instance, someone might think that the life of an embryo or foetus (or some particular embryos or foetuses) is far more important than the life of a pregnant woman (or of a particular pregnant woman) and yet think that abortion should be legal. One might come to this view for various possible reasons. For instance, one might think that it is the job of the state to protect the interests of actual citizens only and that embryos are not actual citizens any more than, say, foxes are. Yet again, one might be in favour of legal abortions, whatever one thinks about the relative moral status and claims of pregnant women and foetuses. This can happen, for example, because of the problems of enforcing laws against abortion. To have laws that are not enforced creates a problem for law and legality in general. If we cannot and/or will not enforce particular laws, then, one might argue, we should not have them and if we do have them, we should repeal them. Do not listen to those who talk about the justification of legislation in terms of 'sending messages'. Laws, rather, send people to prison. Unless one has the stomach to prosecute those who have abortions as criminals, it is unwise to permit abortion to be a crime. I lack such a stomach. That in itself is sufficient for me to be an anti-anti-abortionist whatever I might think about the ethics of having an abortion.

Consider another example. One might argue (as I do and have done) against the invasion of Iraq in 2003 without saying that, or in any way committing one's self to the view that, in a trade-off between the lives of those who would have been killed had an invasion not taken place and the lives of those who were killed as a consequence of the invasion, the latter should be accorded more moral weight. One should not choose to make such a trade-off between people or their lives. The choice between invading and not invading should not have been made on that basis. Nor was this a choice between the moral claims of the one category of people against that of the other despite Harris's analysis of the nature of political decision-making.

It was wrong and unfair of Harris to present Quintavalle's views in the way that he did. Furthermore, Harris has by his misrepresentation confused rather than clarified the issues involved. In his discussion of Quintavalle's alleged position, Harris gives a misleading account of the nature of moral and more particularly political reasoning. He writes:

'This is another example of a case in which we are forced to "trade-off" or choose between moral claims of different groups of people and in which priority is claimed for one side of the equation as against the other. What is required is a genuine and painstaking balance of those competing interests and the costs of prioritising one set over the other'. [3]

Notice, first of all, that this is not actually like what Harris said Quintavalle's position was. To choose between and evaluate claims is not the same as choosing between and evaluating claimants or the lives of claimants. Furthermore, even if decisions sometimes are as Harris outlines them, they are not always like that. We are not invariably forced to make the sort of 'trade-off' that Harris suggests even when decisions involve trade-offs. [6] It is not at all clear that in the case of abortion and of stem-cell research, for example, such a trade-off as Harris suggests is necessary. Who are the 'we' here in Harris's model? This is important. The issue is about the duties of the decision-maker rather than, directly, about the interests and the moral claims of those affected by the decision. Vigilantes, lynch-mobs and assiduous members of kangaroo courts can perform such mental moral arithmetic as Harris talks of: that does not justify their subsequent actions.

The debate over the ethics of, for example, abortion and of stem-cell research might overlap with the debate over the appropriateness of legislation concerning them, but it has a different focus. Should abortion be a crime in the contemporary UK? If so, under what particular circumstances? These questions are not properly answerable by the sort of painstaking calculations that Harris talks of. Should euthanasia be a crime? If so under what circumstances? Should stem-cell research be legal? The same can be said of these questions. There are some kinds of considerations that ought not to determine, perhaps ought not even to influence the particular decisions of particular agents and agencies. Often, we are duty-bound to do certain things whatever the effect is in particular cases. What we should do is to mind our own business relative to the capacity in which we are acting. To keep our attention from the 'big picture' and to ignore our 'values' and 'moral visions' is often our painful duty particularly if we are acting in an official capacity such as a university lecturer marking an examination script or as a Prime Minister contemplating the invasion of Iraq.

*By Hugh V. McLachlan, from *Human Reproduction and Genetic Ethics*, 2006, Vol. 12, No.2.

References

1 Harris JM. Before Birth – After Death *Journal of Medical Ethics* 2004; **30**:425.

2 See, for instance, McLachlan HV. Human Embryos, Clones and Public Policy: A Critique of the Church of Scotland's Views. *Scottish Affairs* 2004; **46**: 110-130.

3 Harris JM. Before Birth – After Death *Journal of Medical Ethics* 2004; **30**:425.
4 McLachlan HV. *Social Justice, Human Rights and Public Policy* Glasgow: Humming Earth, 2005.
5 'Scientists given cloning go ahead'. BBC NEWS, http://news.bbc.co.uk/go/pr/fr/-/hi/health/3554474.shtm
6 See reference 3:13.

Chapter Four

Warnock and Research on Human Embryos: A Case for a Re-Appraisal of the Human Fertilisation and Embryology Act (1990)*

As Sir Anthony Alment has indicated: "Much of the public debate which followed publication of the report of the Committee of Inquiry into Human fertilisation and embryology in July 1984 has followed predictable polarities". (Alment, 1985, p.300)
One such polarity which he highlights is a gradualist view of the development of human life. This is contrasted with what one might call an "absolutist" view of human life. Alment writes:

"Gradualism at the outset of life is naturally rejected by those whose principles hold all life inviolable, and who would, therefore, wish to see present abortion legislation rescinded". (1985, p.302)

I shall comment on this distinction and suggest it is a potentially misleading one. Specifically, I suggest that the arguments presented in the Warnock report concerning the morality of potentially fatal research on human embryos are over-simplified and dogmatic. Consequently, a case for reconsidering the wisdom of the legislation which was enacted on the basis of the acceptance of this report can be established.

Absolutism might be considered as the view that, at conception, a being is created which should be afforded the same moral consideration as any normal human being. In the report, the absolutist's case is presented as follows:

"The human embryo is seen as having the same status as a child or an adult by virtue of its potential for human life. The right to life is held to be the fundamental human right, and the taking of human life on this view is always abhorrent". (Warnock, 1984, p.61).

For at least some absolutists, research on a human embryo seems never to be morally justifiable since it will result in its death. A contrary position might be considered as gradualism. According to the report:

"Others, while in no way denying that human embryos are alive, (and they would concede that eggs and sperm are also alive) hold that embryos are not yet human persons and that if it could be decided when an embryo becomes a person, it could also be decided when it might or might not be permissible for research to be undertaken". (Warnock, 1984, p.60)

The majority of the committee adopted a gradualist approach. They considered that research on a human embryo is not immoral within a particular period of its development but that, thereafter, it should be a criminal offence. The central majority conclusion concerning embryology is that:

"One reference point in the development of the human individual is the formation of the primitive streak. Most authorities put this at about fifteen days after fertilisation. This marks the beginning of individual development of the embryo.... We have therefore regarded an earlier date than this as a desirable end-point for research. We accordingly recommend that no live human embryo derived from in vitro fertilisation, whether frozen or unfrozen, may be kept alive, if not transferred to a woman, beyond that limit of time". (Warnock, 1984, p.66).

Both these views seem to suggest that the central and, perhaps, even the only issue concerning the morality of research on human embryos is the question of when an embryo becomes a human person. The absolutists and the gradualist differ only in offering differing answers to it. However, the question is wrongly framed and to direct attention towards it serves to over-simplify a complex moral issue. In one clear sense, a human embryo cannot be considered as a person. An embryo never becomes a person. An embryo is a partially developed form of what might become the body of a person. It is to *persons* rather than their *bodies* that moral respect is due. We have moral duties towards the persons rather than towards bodies, although we have duties concerning peoples' bodies. Similarly, persons rather than bodies are the bearers of moral rights.

If an embryo cannot be considered as a person, does it follow that moral considerations need not circumscribe our behaviour towards it? Does it follow that the question of the ethics of research on human embryos produced *in vitro* is morally a non-issue? I think that the correct answer to both questions is: no.

Suppose that one were to accept the contentious propositions that moral respect is due only to human persons. Does it follow that such respect must be shown only to persons who have *currently living* bodies? This would seem to me to be an arbitrary restriction. Consider, for instance, the dead. It does not seem unreasonable to say that we have duties concerning such people and, in some case, duties towards them in the sense that, although no longer possessing living human bodies, they have rights against us. I think this is one reason why we feel obliged to take heed of people's wills even if we are not always able to carry them out to the letter. We often feel obliged to adopt conservation policies. Does this not suggest that we feel we have duties concerning and/or towards future generations or, towards persons who do not have currently living human bodies? Would it not be immoral if we were to wantonly and knowingly pollute the planet in such a way that it would be uninhabitable in, say, one hundred years' time, even if relatively comfortable until then? If this would be immoral, then it would seem to follow that moral respect is not due solely to persons with living bodies (See McLachlan, 1976 and 1977).

Rather than talk of moral respect for embryos and of the rights of embryos and of our moral duties towards and concerning them, it seems to me to be more sensible to talk of moral respect for the persons into whose living human bodies such embryos might develop and of their rights and of our duties towards and concerning them. If we re-address the issue in this way then, of course, we will still be faced with the difficult judgement of whether in particular cases research on a human embryo is morally justifiable or desirable. However, I think that we will be less likely to accept the rigid conclusions of either the absolutism or gradualism which we have been discussing.

Consider first of all the gradualism of the majority conclusion. If moral respect is due to a person into whose body an embryo might develop, then any moral responsibilities or obligations which we might have do not, somehow, emerge at a particular stage of the embryo's development. Suppose that a particular embryo has developed *in vitro* for, say, eight days. Is it morally justifiable to conduct research on it? It seems to me that, *in abstracto,* no categorical answers can be given to questions such as: What is the likely outcome of the research? What is the likely fate of the embryo if research is not carried out on it? There might be barren women who would be desperately keen to have it implanted in their wombs in the likelihood of its successful delivery. Would such implantation be morally preferable to experimentation and, if so, would it follow that the experimentation would be morally unjustifiable or wrong? The situation would seem more clear-cut if the embryo was a "spare" one, i.e. in addition to requirements for implantation. Here one might well argue that since, left *in vitro,* the embryo will die anyway, nothing is lost and something might be gained by conducting research on it. Nonetheless, it might be countered that it is not clear-cut whether or not a particular embryo is "spare". It depends, for instance, on how hard we try to find and encourage recipients and on how long we, say, keep an embryo in a frozen state for possible future recipients. Suppose that a particular embryo has developed *in vitro* for, say, 20 days. It does not seem to me that it would always be immoral to conduct research on it. Suppose that if, for whatever reasons, it was not possible or practical to store or implant it. Why would it be wrong to conduct research on it? Who would suffer from it?

The view of the majority of the committee seems to be that it is not immoral and should not be illegal to conduct potentially fatal research on an *in vitro* embryo which has developed for fourteen days or less since such an embryo is not an individual human being. Thereafter, they consider that such an embryo is, or might be, an individual human being and consequently, not only must no research be carried out on it, but it must not be kept alive. It is difficult to make sense of this latter conclusion, even in terms of the language and *rationale* of the report. In what sense can the injunction not to keep such an embryo alive be thought to protect "the embryo" as the report claims? Who benefits from it? I think that, in their own terms, the majority would have been more consistent to say that, since the embryo which has developed more than fourteen days is an individual human being, every reasonable effort should be made to keep it alive whether *in vitro* or whatever. However, they explicitly state their conviction that the production of an *in vitro* child should be a criminal offence (See Warnock, 1984, pp.71-72). This seems to me to be most curious. How does the recommendation protect the interests of the persons into whose mature bodies such embryos might have developed?

The majority of the committee seem to turn the notion of a "right to life" on its head. The claim, that an embryo which has developed for more than fourteen days should not be kept alive *in vitro,* might be ambiguous. Perhaps, the claim is merely that such embryos should be *allowed* to die, that no efforts should be made to keep them alive. However the suggestion seems to be stronger than this. It is re-stated as: " ... our recommendation is that the growing of a human embryo *in vitro* beyond fourteen days should be a criminal offence" (Warnock, 1984, p. 72). The suggestion seems to be that such embryos should be killed. It is a long way from saying that one has a "right to life" to saying that one or another has a duty to kill particular embryos.

Mention of a "right to life" brings us back to a consideration of absolutism. According to the absolutist, people have a "right to life", and, according to them, to conduct potentially fatal research on an embryo is equivalent to performing such research on adults and children. It is further suggested that: "Everyone agrees that it is completely unacceptable to make use of a child or an adult as the subject of a research procedure which may cause harm or death" (Warnock, 1984, p.61). It behoves one who wants to argue that research on human embryos might in some circumstances be morally justified, as I do, either to claim that such research on an adult or child might sometimes be justified or to suggest wherein lies the difference.

First of all, let us consider in what sense people might be thought to have a "right to life". There are at least two clear senses in which we talk of "rights", namely, rights of action correspond to absences of obligation. We might say that we have, for instance, a right of action to marry a particular girl or to pick a particular wild fruit in that we are not obliged not to. Of course, other people will have the same rights of action and if they exercise them before we do, we are likely not to be in a position to exercise ours. It would seem uncontroversial to say that we have a right to life in the sense that we are not obliged not to live, but nothing would seem to follow from this regarding how we should behave towards other people or embryos. On the other hand, rights of recipience correspond to other people's duties. The most obvious examples are contractual or quasi – contractual ones. For instance, if a friend borrows my lawnmower, then I have the right to its return not only in the sense that I am under no obligation not to re-acquire it, but in the sense that my friend has a duty to return it to me. My right to receive the lawnmower corresponds to his or her duty. To call something a "human" right is presumably to appeal to the tradition of natural law theory according to which human beings by virtue of being human beings, have particular moral rights against and duties towards all other human beings. It has traditionally been argued that people have a right of (negative) recipience to life in the sense that, regarding any one person, all others have a duty not to kill him or her.

Is it plausible to argue that people have a natural right of positive recipience to life? I do not think that it is. It might be plausible to say that I and all other members of the human race have a duty not to kill another since, apart from anything else, it is physically possible to fulfil such a duty. However, it does not make sense to say that I have a natural duty to feed, clothe and provide any other necessities of life for all other people and that, correspondingly, of natural right, I can demand that all others do the same for me.

Nonetheless, might it not be argued that we have a moral duty to do all that we can to try to promote human life even if no-one is a bearer of a corresponding right? I think there are problems with such a claim. There is a difference between saying that a particular course of action is morally laudable and saying that it is morally obligatory. Failure to live like, say, Mother Theresa, is not necessarily to neglect one's moral duties. Furthermore, there is the problem of deciding what particular human lives to promote. After all, Mother Theresa could work in Ethiopia, say, rather than India. The money raised by Live-Aid could be used in India rather than Ethiopia, or used to finance cancer research, and so on and so forth. Lastly, even if we do have a duty to promote life, this might clash with other duties. For instance, suppose that we have, among other choices, the choice between giving more to try to feed some starving people or giving more to try to comfort and alleviate the pain of the terminally ill and some other such tormented people. Is it always, or ever, clear in such circumstances what morally we ought to do?

Suppose that someone is in hospital with heart, kidney and lung failure and in a coma which in the normal way of things would be irreversible. Now, it might be possible to prolong the person's life through a series of expensive operations, and in some circumstances this might be the appropriate thing to do, although it is not clear to me that the person has a *right* to such treatment in the sense that any individual or collectively is the bearer of a corresponding duty. Suppose it is decided not to perform the operation. For the sake of simplicity, suppose that the requisite organs for transplantation are unavailable and that it is known that without them the patient will die in a matter of hours. Suppose that it were possible to conduct some research on the person's body which would hasten his or her demise but would be useful in improving the health of and increasing the life-span of other people. Would it always be morally wrong to perform such research? It is not clear to me that it always would be wrong and, if so, why would it be wrong. It would seem to me to be rather weak to say that it is wrong because the person has a right of negative recipience to live since, in the example, this is not one which he or she is in a position to benefit from. Of course, one might hold the view that, while such research is not always immoral, it should always be illegal, but that is another matter. One might argue that the possibility of the practice might lead to abuses and that living people might be experimented on who actually would otherwise have survived. In addition, knowledge of the practice might well cause concern to potential and actual hospital patients, especially those of a suspicious nature.

Suppose that an embryo is developing *in vitro.* In some circumstances, it might be appropriate and even generous to try and foster its development, perhaps especially if a woman is willing to receive it in her womb, even although no-one or other has a duty to ensure that this takes place and no-one holds the right of recipience to such treatment. Nevertheless, there might well be circumstances where there is no such willing woman and no-one willing and/or able to store or otherwise tend the embryo. In circumstances where the embryo is bound to die anyway even if research is not conducted upon it, it seems to me that such research might be justifiable even if this were to be thought to disregard the right to life of the person concerned. Such research is different from research on normal healthy adults and children since, generally, we can reasonably assume that, if we do not perform such research, then they will continue to live and experience life. It is for this reason that, for them, the right of negative recipience to live is an important one.

According to the Committee's absolutist dissenters, while embryos might be produced *in vitro,* research should never be carried out upon them. They write:

"In the event of there being more embryos than is judged right to implant at any one time the remainder should either be frozen with a view to implantation at a later date or allowed to die. They should not be used for experimentation. Still less should embryos be deliberately created for the purpose of experimentation". (Warnock, 1984, pp. 91-92).

Two paradoxical features of the dissenters' case spring to mind. They are adamant that embryos should not be deliberately created for experimentation. However, if these particular embryos are not created for experimentation, they will not be created at all. It might seem curious to say that, in defence of the right of life, such embryos should not be created especially since, after all, some embryos deliberately created for research purposes might actually end up being implanted. Who would benefit from the injunction not to create such embryos?

The dissenters write: "Because embryos have the potential to become human persons neither the relief of infertility nor the advance of knowledge justifies their deliberate destruction". (Warnock, 1984, p.92)
Suppose that such research did increase human fertility. Then, people who otherwise would not have been born might well not only possess but be in a position to enjoy the right to life. Again, it is curious to want to rule out such a possibility by appealing to a relatively trivial instance of a right to life of negative recipience.

The moral issues involved in embryology are less straight-forward and clear-cut than the report allows. Both those who oppose research on human embryos and those who, within limits do not oppose it – what we might call the absolutists and the gradualists respectively – present the issue in a misleadingly over-simplified way. They both focus their attention on the question of when, if at all, an embryo becomes a person and differ largely in offering different answers to it. Whether potentially fatal research on an embryo or any other human body is morally justified is not solely dependent on the age or state of development of the body concerned. Of course, the question of whether and when such research should be illegal even if it is not immoral and, indeed, whether and when it should be legal, even if it is immoral, remains an open one. Although they are provocative, the deliberations of the Warnock committee provide an inadequate basis for answering it (See McLachlan, 1985).

I do not want to suggest that the Warnock Report provided all the arguments on the grounds of which the Human Fertilisation and Embryology Act (1990) was framed and passed: nor do I suggest that this legislation is necessarily defective in every detail, nevertheless, given that the report was explicitly commissioned in the contemplation of legislation in this area, the fact that the argumentation of the report is so defective gives us reason and should give us a cause for reconsidering the Act. In particular, I think we should re-assess the *rationale* for the following provisions of the Act. First of all, there is the stipulation that "A licence cannot authorise – (a) keeping or using an embryo after the appearance of the primitive streak..." (3) Secondly, that: "A woman shall not be provided with any treatment or services involving – (b) the use of any embryo the creation of which was brought about *in vitro ...*" (6) Thirdly, the specification "...that no gametes or embryos shall be kept in storage for longer than the statutory storage period, and, if stored at the end of the period, shall be allowed to perish..." (14c) – must not be allowed to live? – seems to be an especially heinous one.

*By Hugh V. McLachlan, *International Journal of Sociology and Social Policy*, Vol. 13, No. 5/6, pp. 110-119

Bibliography

1. Alment, Sir Anthony, (1985) *Contemporary Review.*
2. McLachlan, H.V. (1985) "In Defence of Surrogate Motherhood". *Contemporary Review* January.
3. McLachlan, H. V. (1976) "Moral Rights and Abortion". *Contemporary Review.*
4. McLachlan, H. V. (1977) "Must we Accept Either the Conservative or Liberal View on Abortion?" *Analysis* Vol. 37, No. 4.
5. Warnock, M. (1984) *Report of the Committee of Inquiry into Human Fertilisation and Embryology.* Chairperson, Dame Mary Warnock, July 1984. Her Majesty's Stationery Office, Cmnd. 9314.

Chapter Five

Persons and Their Bodies: How We Should Think About Human Embryos*

Abstract

The status of human embryos is discussed particularly in the light of the claim by Fox, in Health Care Analysis 8 that it would be useful to think of them in terms of cyborg metaphors. It is argued that we should consider human embryos for what they are – partially formed human bodies – rather than for what they are like in some respects (and unlike in others) – cyborgs. However to settle the issue of the status of the embryo is not to answer the moral questions which arise concerning how embryos should be treated. Since persons rather than bodies have rights, embryos do not have rights. However, whether or not embryos have rights, people can have duties concerning them. Furthermore, the persons whose fully developed bodies embryos will, might (or might have) become can have rights. Contrary to what is often assumed, it is not merely persons who have (or have had) living, developed human bodies who have moral rights: so it is argued in this paper.

Key words: *bodies, cyborgs, embryos, fetuses, persons, property, rights*

Introduction

In a recent article, Fox argues that the usual ways of talking and thinking about human embryos are unsatisfactory. She writes: "While conceding that the issue of embryo status is essentially contestable ..., this essay has argued for the need [to] introduce new ways in which to conceptualise the embryo, avoiding the unsatisfactory person/ property dichotomy" (Fox, 2000: 184).

I shall comment on Fox's views. I shall contend that, in the context of embryology, the relationships between property, rights, persons, and bodies should be reconsidered but not precisely in the particular way which Fox suggests. No new terminology is required. We can use old ways of talking to say new or different things.

Fox's Position

The usual approach, Fox says, has been to start from the assumption that embryos must be either persons or else property but then to conclude that embryos have some sort of status mid-way between that of persons and property. Fox contends that: "Significantly, designating the embryo as halfway between person and property reflects the approach of Warnock and the Bioethics convention, and is indicative of an emerging international consensus on the legal status of embryo[s]" (Fox, 2000: 181).

This designation is, according to Fox, a fudge. Fox writes: "Even if researchers are comfortable with such a fudge, I would argue that such a position is unsatisfactory and leads to difficulty in resolving more recent debates over the ethics of cloning embryos" (Fox, 2000: 184).

She writes too:

"I argue that it might be productive to shift the debate from this polarised dispute over whether embryos matter or not, whether they are pre-persons or commodities. Instead, I suggest that we should attempt to locate them in a biotechnological milieu, where cyborg metaphors might be utilised, and questions of how we should treat embryos would be contextualised alongside our responses to other cyborgs" (Fox, 2000: abstract, 171).

The Usual Approach to the Classification of Embryos

It is not clear that Fox is correct in maintaining that the embryo actually is commonly considered to be mid-way between being a person and being property. Secondly, it is not clear that the attribution of such a borderline status would necessarily, *per se,* be a fudge: some phenomena are, given the logic of classificatory schemes, borderlines and the rational thing to do is to consider them as such.

Consider an analogy. Not everything – and, indeed, not even every person – is either male or female. (The term 'he or she' does not actually succeed in being totally inclusive. For the politically correct, 'he, she, it or whatever' would be a more apt term.) Some things – and some people – are neither male nor female. A eunuch, for instance, is neither male nor female and is, perhaps, a borderline male but is not midway between being a male and being a female. Some people – hermaphrodites – are both male and female: that is not the same as being midway between being male and female. The red *Chambers Dictionary* which lies before me on my desk is, like my desk, neither male nor female and nor is it mid-way between being male and female.

The categories 'person' and 'property' are not dichotomous ones any more than are the categories 'male' and 'female'. People and things cannot be classified *exhaustively* as either 'persons' or 'property'. Fox is wrong, I think, when she says: "Currently, I would argue that dominant legal constructions of the embryo/foetus are premised on a personhood/ property binary" (Fox, 2000: 172).

It seems to me that British and other legal jurisdictions do not consider that everything is either a person or else property. Many things are neither persons nor property. For instance, although you and I are persons, our bodies are, obviously, not persons. However, it does not follow that our bodies are property (see McLachlan, 1997). Some parts of them might be property but not all parts of them are property. For instance, if I entered into an agreement with someone to sell to him my living heart and brain, no court in the land would honour such an arrangement. Courts, however, might honour an agreement for the sale of, say, a lock of my hair. Similarly our bodies as such are not property. Our own bodies are not our property and neither are they anyone else's property. Our bodies are not midway between being person's and being property: they belong to neither of these categories and nor are they located between them. They are other than persons or property.

I am not sure what sense, if any, it makes to talk of a status *between* property and personhood. The 'property'/'person' distinction is not an exhaustive nor dichotomous one and nor is it a polar distinction. A town, for instance, might be borderline-French and, say, borderline-German but nothing is in the same sense borderline-person and borderline-property because, whereas France and Germany are spatially contiguous, 'person' and 'property' are not, so to speak, conceptually contiguous. They do not merge: they are different types of categories from each other; they are not, as it were, at either ends of the same continuum.

Consider an example that is cited by Fox herself in her article. The Supreme Court of Tennessee, so Fox tell us, held that:

" '...pre-embryos are not, strictly speaking, either 'persons' or 'property', but occupy an interim category that entitled them to special respect because of their potential for human life'. It noted that the interest was not a true property interest but was akin to 'the nature of ownership, to the extent that [the progenitors have] decision-making authority concerning the disposition of the pre-embryos' " (Fox, 2000: 180).

Despite what Fox says, this does not 'fudge' the issue. This addresses the issue in a non-fudged way and gives an eminently reasonable interpretation of it. Fetuses are unusual sorts of things and have, understandably, an unusual legal status. So this legal judgement seems to say: it claims that a fetus is not a person or property; it claims that it is like property without being property – borderline property, perhaps. It does not claim that fetuses have a status midway between property and personhood.

Warnock and the Status of Human Embryos

Reading the Warnock Report, I cannot discover the suggested view that embryos have a status midway between that of being property and being persons. I can find suggestions of what the legal status of fetuses should be - not all of them coherent nor, perhaps, mutually consistent – but I cannot find that particular view.

It says in the Warnock Report that, although they should not have the same status as adults or children, human embryos should have "a special status" in law and that they "*... should be afforded some protection in law*" (Warnock, 1985: 63). Warnock goes on to say: "*We accordingly recommend that no live human embryo derived from in vitro fertilisation, whether frozen or unfrozen, may be kept alive, if not transferred to a woman, beyond fourteen days after fertilization ...*" (Warnock, 1985: 66).

This is a bizarre way to 'protect' the embryo! The embryo, in the situation described here, must not be allowed to live: it must be killed. I hope that Warnock and her committee do not try to 'protect' me and my family if this is an indication of what their protection can involve (see McLachlan, 1993, 1995).

Bizarre this might be, but it is not the suggestion that embryos are midway between property and personhood. It is explicitly said in the Warnock Report that embryos should *not* be treated as property. However, subsequent statements made in the Report might be thought to water down and qualify this strong proposal. One reads in the Report: "The concept of ownership of human embryos seems to us undesirable. *We recommend that legislation be enacted to ensure there is no right to ownership in a human embryo* (Warnock, 1985: 56).

However, in the very next sentence, it says:

"Nevertheless, the couple who have stored an embryo for their use should be recognised as having rights to the use and disposal of the embryo, although these rights ought to be subject to limitation ... *We therefore recommend that when one of a couple dies the right to use or dispose o[f] any embryo stored by that couple should pass to the survivor .... We recommend that if both die that right should pass to the storage authority*" (Warnock, 1985: 56).

Do such rights of disposal and control amount, despite what is said in the previously quoted sentence, to the classification of embryos as property? I do not think so. Not all rights are property rights. Not all rights concerning disposal and control are property rights. There is a difference between *having* rights of disposal and control and *owning* them. Hence, it does not follow that if people have rights regarding the control and disposal of embryos, embryos are property. For instance, I not only *have* particular rights of disposal and control concerning my house, I *own* them. I can sell them or give them away. (Such rights of disposal, control and voluntary transfer are not absolute nor without qualification. It is a childish fallacy that one can do what one wants with one's own property or, for that matter, with one's own body (see McLachlan, 1997)). Parents *have* particular rights concerning the disposal and control of their children which the rest of us do not have concerning these particular children. However, the parents do not *own* these rights. Neither the rights nor the children *are property*. Neither the rights nor the children can be sold or given away as gifts.

However, the following suggestion in the Warnock report seems to me to involve regarding embryos as property or, at least, as borderline-property. There will be transactions between licensed agencies. What if there is to be a transfer of gametes and embryos between them? The report says:

"... a complete prohibition on the purchase or sale of such material would be inappropriate. A balance has to be struck and therefore *we recommend that the sale or purchase of human gametes or embryos should be permitted only under licence from, and subject to, conditions prescribed by the licensing body and therefore unauthorised sale or purchase should be made a criminal offence*" (Warnock, 1985: 79).

The Warnock Report might be interpreted here as suggesting that while embryos should not be the property of individual people, they could be the property of particular sorts of agencies or institutions. As is always the case, the rights involved are limited and qualified and they are accompanied by property duties.

Rights, Bodies and Persons

Particularly with reference to abortion, some people talk about the rights and/or the lack of rights of fetuses (see McLachlan, 1977). This is very curious. A fetus is a partially developed human body (just as an embryo is a human body in an even less advanced stage of development). It might or might not become a mature human body. Human arms and legs do not have rights. Human bodies – no matter the state of their development – do not have rights. Persons have rights. They have rights to and concerning their arms, legs and their bodies but not merely to nor concerning them.

Bodies do not have rights. Embryos are partially formed bodies. Embryos have no rights. Of course, to say that embryos have no rights is not to close the ethical discussion of the treatment of – including, for instance, the issue of research on – human embryos. For instance, trees do not have rights but it does not follow that we are entitled to treat them any way we like. We can have duties concerning, say, trees, animals and embryos whether or not trees, animals and embryos have rights.

Furthermore, even if it is persons (and not bodies) who have moral rights, it does not follow that only persons whose bodies are currently developed and alive have moral rights. I would say that while embryos do not have moral rights, the person into whose mature human body an embryo might develop (or might have developed) can have moral rights. The possession of a currently living body – whether or not a developed one – is not a necessary feature for the possession of moral rights.

It seems to be the view of, for instance, Brazier, Campbell and Golombok, as expressed in their Report on Surrogate Motherhood, that only people who have bodies which are currently alive have moral rights and/or are due moral consideration (see Brazier *et al.*, 1998). Campbell persists with the assertion of the view (although he fails to support it) in his debate with Harris on 'the welfare of the child' (see Campbell, 2000; Harris, 2000).

Perhaps the only persons who have *legal* rights are those who have (or those who have and those who have had) living human bodies. That is a different issue and one I shall not explore here. Perhaps too, at least in some instances, the moral rights of those who have living human bodies might be stronger than those of other people and they might be different from the rights of other people. However, people who do not have human bodies which are currently alive can be due moral consideration and they can, moreover, have moral rights.

Consider some examples. Suppose that I promise to a friend that I will, say, look after his cat and tend his garden should he become unable to do so himself. I thereby create a duty for me to do these things and a right for him that, under specified circumstances, these things are done by me. Suppose that my friend were to die. My duty would not die with him and nor, I would say, would his right. Even if my friend no longer had a living human body, that person, I would say, would still have rights. He would have, for instance, the right to my conscientious endeavour to ensure that his cat is cared for and his garden is tended by me.

If you are uneasy with the notion of a deceased person still possessing rights – and the unease, I suggest, is misplaced – then, surely, you would at least allow that I, the promisor, can have duties *concerning* him. I have, after all, duties concerning my friend's cat and garden even although my friend's cat and my friend's garden do not have currently living human bodies. Even if I had not made the promise, I would still have duties, even if different ones, to and concerning his cat and garden. For instance, we all have, an obligation, for instance, not to torture cats and not to despoil gardens.

If we were to obliterate today the planet earth, then there are innumerable people who would otherwise have had living human bodies who would not come to have them. I suggest not only that we have duties concerning these people but that these people are (today) the bearers of rights against us. What precisely the rights and duties are is a question which I will avoid here. I am not suggesting (nor do I hold) an extreme environmentalist position nor anything like it. I want merely to assert that – however weak or strong they might be – there are such duties and rights concerning and enjoyed by people who do not have currently living bodies and who have not had and who might never have living human bodies.

In the moral and legal sense of the term one can enjoy rights which one does not enjoy in the psychological sense of the term. One can have particular moral and legal rights which one does not need, want and/or benefit from while one is alive: consequently, that one does not want, need nor benefit from rights when one is not alive would not be a reason for saying that one does not have rights when one is not alive.

My View Contrasted with One Expressed in the Warnock Report

It might help to clarify my view to contrast it with the following one. This is a view expressed in but not necessarily the view of the Warnock Report:

'At one end is the proposition that it is only *to human persons* that respect must be accorded. A human embryo cannot be thought of as a person, or even as a potential person. It is simply a collection of cells which, unless it implants in a human uterine environment, has no potential for development. There is no reason to accord these cells any protected status' (Warnock, 1985: 62).

Let us breakdown and number some of the propositions here.

1) ... it is only to *human persons* that respect must be

accorded.

2) A human embryo cannot be thought of as a person, or even as a potential person.

3) It is simply a collection of cells which, unless it implants in a human uterine environment, has no potential for development.

4) There is no reason to accord these cells any protected status.

I would say that (1) and (4) are false but (2) is true. (3) is partly true: an embryo is a collection of cells but it is not 'simply' a collection of cells; it might become (or could have become) the developed human body of a person. This is a sufficient reason – (4) is false – for according it respect although it is not a necessary condition for according it respect: (1) is also false. Such things as, for instance, trees, paintings, buildings, including but not merely listed ones, my (and other people's) cats, the truth, and the Scottish Football Association must be accorded respect. (How much? and in what contexts? are matters of legitimate debate.)

It is persons rather than the bodies of persons who are the bearers of rights and duties (although agencies such as, say, Elderslie Golf Club and Glasgow Caledonian University as well as agents such as you and I can and do have moral and legal rights and duties). My arms, say, and your arms have no rights or duties. Our bodies have no rights or duties. We as persons have rights and duties including those concerning our own and other people's bodies. For instance, we have a duty to keep our own bodies clean and, in many contexts, clothed. We have duties towards the bodies of others which correspond to rights they have concerning their own bodies. For instance, we have a duty, while they are yet alive at least, not deliberately to set them on fire. We have a duty not to collide with them avoidably when we are driving our motor cars as well as various other duties concerning the bodies of other people. Although the bodies of other people are, obviously, not persons, they must be treated with respect.

Conclusion

Let us think about and talk about embryos as what they are rather than what they are not or than what they are like – as least as a starting-point. I think that the cyborg metaphor, like any other metaphor, is an unreliable *basis* for thought:

A metaphor, to quote my *Chambers English Dictionary* is "... a figure of speech by which a thing is spoken of as being that which it only resembles, as when a ferocious man is called a tiger". To call a man a tiger might be illuminating for some purposes but it is false. However, if one were to use a simile rather than a metaphor and say that a man, or a particular one, is *like* a tiger, then one can retain the illuminating effect of the figure of speech and also speak truly. One can speak just as truly and more specifically if one says that so and so is like a tiger with respect to ferocity (but not – perhaps – very, very much). Similarly, one might say that an embryo is like a cyborg and then go on to specify the respect and, possibly, the extent of the similarity. However, let us start with a consideration of what embryos are. Without that, the aptness and truthfulness of figures of speech as applied to embryos cannot be appraised.

Whether the embryo is considered as a person or property is not the pivotal issue. Failure to regard it as the pivotal issue is not to duck or fudge it. An embryo is neither a person nor (unequivocally) property. It could become (unequivocally) property if our legal conventions and interpretations of them changed. It could not become a person. Likewise, my *Chambers Dictionary* could not become a person.

What is contestable is not so much the status of the embryo but the relevance of the status of the embryo. Embryos are partially formed human bodies. I am not sure that this claimed status of the embryo is 'essentially contestable'. It seems, rather, undeniable. It seems undeniable too that, while persons can *have,* for instance, minds, personalities and bodies, bodies *are not* persons. *A fortiori,* partially formed bodies are not persons: nor are they partially formed persons.

There is no 'person/property dichotomy' to avoid. There is a distinction between persons and property but not an exhaustive nor dichotomous one. Furthermore, the question of whether something is or is not property is, perhaps, wrongly put. The unauthorised sale and purchase of, say, heroin, is a criminal offence. Does it follow that heroin in not property? I don't know. One can have rights concerning the disposal and control of heroin which are other than property rights even when (as when it is prescribed for one) the heroin might be thought of – but perhaps wrongly? – as one's own property. Hospitals and pharmacies can sell heroin but only under certain conditions and only to certain parties.

The salient question is not whether or not, say, heroin or embryos are property. One should, rather, ask: what property rights and duties does one have in relation to them?; what non-property rights and duties does one have in relation to them?

I stress the duties as much as the rights: there is a danger of thinking wrongly of property relations solely in terms of rights. Sometimes, the rights of property ownership are slight and unavailing while the duties are burdensome and highly restrictive. If embryos, or some of them, became property it does not follow that wanton and inappropriate treatment of them would become permissible and/or more likely. Consider, for instance, cats. Some cats are and some cats are not the property of specific people. It is far from clear that the latter cats are treated better than the former cats. It is far from clear that worse treatment of the former cats than the latter cats is legally permitted.

One is not necessarily permitted to treat a cat which one owns in the same ways that one might treat an 'X' which one owns. It depends what 'X' stands for. Different instances of property relationships can involve different clusters of rights and duties. To say that one owns an 'X' – say, an embryo is to leave pretty much open the question of the nature and content of the cluster of rights and duties involved. One might own, say, a lump of coal and a cat. Is one permitted, say, to set fire to such property of one's own? It depends. If the cat is dead, one might, if it is safe to do so, set it on fire. One might not set the coal on fire, whether it is safe to do so or not, if one lives in Britain in certain specified areas.

Concerns about property relationships and 'commodification' in relation to, for instance, embryos, babies, prostitutes, and commercial surrogate mothers, often arise from misunderstandings about the nature of property and ownership (see McLachlan and Swales, 2000).

*By Hugh V. McLachlan, from *Health Care Analysis*, 2002, Vol. 10, No. 2, pp. 155-164. With kind permission of Springer Sciences and Business Media.

References

Brazier, M, Campbell, A, and Golombok, S. (1998) *Surrogacy: Review for Health Ministers of Current Arrangements for Payments and Regulations; Report of the Review Team.* CM 4068.

Campbell, A.V. (2000) Surrogacy, Rights and Duties: A Partial Commentary. *Health Care Analysis* 8, 35-40.

Fox, M. (2000) Pre-Persons, Commodities or Cyborgs: The Legal Construction and Representation of the Embryo. *Health Care Analysis* 8, 171-181.

Harris, J. (2000) The Welfare of the Child. *Health Care Analysis* 8, 27-34.

McLachlan, H.V. (1977) Must We Accept Either the Conservative or the Liberal View on Abortion? *Analysis* 37, 197-204.

McLachlan, H.V. (1993) Warnock and Research on Human Embryos: A Case for a Re-Appraisal of the Fertilisation and Embryology Act (1990). *International Journal of Sociology and Social Policy* **13,**110-119.
McLachlan, H.V. (1995) On Producing Embryos for Research. *The Philosopher* **21,** 2-11.
McLachlan, H.V. (1997) Bodies, Rights and Abortion. *Journal of Medical Ethics* 23, 176-180.
McLachlan, H.V. and Swales, J.K. (2000) Babies, Child Bearers and Commodification: Anderson, Brazier *et al.*, and the Political Economy of Commercial Surrogate Motherhood. *Health Care Analysis* 8, 1-18.
Warnock, M. (1985) A *Question of Life: The Warnock Report on Human Fertilisation and Embryology.* Oxford: Blackwell.

Chapter Six

Human Embryos, Clones and Public Policy: A Critique of the Church of Scotland's Views*

Introduction

I shall discuss some views endorsed by the Church of Scotland on the theology, ethics and the appropriate public policy towards research on human embryos and human cloning. (1) These views are, in essence, that both research on human embryos and the cloning of human beings are contrary to Christianity, are immoral and, most significantly, should be illegal. I shall argue that none of these views is substantiated.

The Views on Embryology and on Research on Human Embryos of the Church of Scotland

The thinking of the Church on human embryos is presented in *Pre-conceived Ideas: A Christian Perspective of IVF and Embryology*, (1996) which is the report of the Study Group on Human Fertilisation and Embryology of the Board of Social Responsibility of the Church of Scotland. (2) The position of the Study Group – as accepted by the General Assembly – is as follows. We should not do research on persons unless it is for their benefit and/or with their consent. The embryo is a person or, at least, (the report is equivocal on this point) a potential person. We should not do research on human embryos unless it is for their benefit (since they cannot give consent). It is, in their view, wrong to do and it should be illegal to do it. The sort of research envisaged will, quite clearly, not be in the interest of the embryos concerned: indeed, it will be, directly or indirectly, fatal for them.

It is written:

'According to the theological and ethical position stated [in the report], the human embryo must be regarded as an actual person, and regarded as a person at all stages of development from the moment of conception. Therefore all treatment of a human embryo which is not for the benefit of that embryo is morally wrong and as such all research on human embryos is morally wrong'. (*Church of Scotland*, 1996, p. 62)

We must, I agree, treat embryos with respect. We should not wantonly create or wantonly destroy them. But to say this is not to say that embryos are persons or that they have rights. After, all, we must respect, for instance, cats, dogs and trees and we have duties concerning these things even if they do not have rights and although they are not persons. (3)

The Study Group gives its views not merely on the theology and ethics of embryology but on public policy regarding it. In the conclusion of their report, it: 'Affirms the sanctity of the human embryo from conception, and urges that its special nature be recognised in law' and: 'Given that the law allows research on human embryos, welcomes the limitation of research to 14 days, and opposes any extension of that limit. (*Church of Scotland*, 1996, p. 81)

An Appraisal of the Kernel of the Church of Scotland's Philosophy of Embryology

The essence of the Church of Scotland's case can be represented as follows:

> A): the embryo is a potential person.
> B): because it is a potential person, the embryo should be treated as if it already were a person.
> C): because fetuses and persons are at different ends of a continuum in which there are no discrete nor distinct cut-off points, fetuses and persons should be treated the same.

Even if A) were true, B) is false and C) is false. However, A) is also false.

First of all, consider C). Consider, for instance, differential treatment with respect to age. In terms of age, all living people are at different points on a continuum in which there are no discrete cut-off points. Nonetheless, it is often ethically appropriate for people to treat other people differently in terms of age even in the absence of unequivocal ethical boundaries. Similarly, it is often appropriate to have legal differences between the treatment of people of different ages even in the absence of unequivocal relevant ethical criteria for discriminating. For instance, it is quite appropriate that people have to be of a certain age before they are allowed to do various things, for instance, to get married, to vote in general elections, to purchase tobacco, to purchase alcohol and to drive heavy goods vehicles. The age need not, of course, be the same for all the activities. Similarly, it need not be the same for all people for each of the particular activities but there are obvious practical advantages in making it the same.

Should the age when people are allowed to marry be, say, 17

years? Why should it be 17 rather than 17 and a half years or 17 years and three quarters? Why should it be 17 years rather than 16 years and 364 days? What ethical landmark is passed after one more day? None at all. It is crucially important that a line is drawn somewhere. It is not crucially important precisely where it is drawn. It might be crucially important where, vaguely, the line is drawn.

Wherever the line is drawn, it will, in relation to the maturity of some particular young people, be set at too old an age and, in relation to the immaturity of some other particular young people, it will be set at too young an age. Lines often must be drawn somewhere. The absence of specific ethical criteria should not, in all cases, prevent the drawing of legal lines. C) is false.

Even if there were no laws against having sex with very young people, it would still be immoral to do so. It would be – quite clearly! – wrong in all cases for people over, say, twenty years of age to have sexual intercourse with, say, seven – year-olds. However, would it be immoral in all cases for them to have sex with people aged virtually but not quite eighteen, seventeen, fifteen or sixteen years? I don't know. Ethically, distinctions must be made and, often, one must discriminate even in the absence of obvious moral landmarks.

According to the report:

'The embryo contains within its genetic code all that is needed to become a person. Only its development is necessary. That development is to be seen not as a growth into that which it was not before, but rather as the fulfilment of that which it already is. There is therefore continuity of identity from zygote to fetus, from fetus to new-born child, and from new-born child to adult.' (*Church of Scotland*, 1996, p. 56)

Particular tadpoles, if they develop normally, turn into particular frogs. There is thus, in a sense, a continuity of identity between tadpoles and frogs. However, there are manifest differences between tadpoles and frogs, including between particular frogs which were once particular tadpoles. We are not required by reason nor morality to treat tadpoles as if they were frogs nor frogs as if they were really tadpoles. One might, without acting wrongly or absurdly, treat frogs and tadpoles differently and treat frogs as if they were frogs and tadpoles as if they were tadpoles. Similarly, it is not a requirement of reason or morality or of Christianity that one treats human adults as if they were human embryos or human embryos as if they were, say, babies or children. Ashes to ashes, dust to dust – there is, of course, a continuity, but the differences matter too and matter hugely.

In any case, it is false to say that embryos contain within their genetic code all that is needed to become persons. A) is false. Embryos are not potential persons: they are actual undeveloped human bodies and potential mature human bodies. Bodies are not persons. (See McLachlan, 2002a and 2002b) Persons can have bodies but bodies are not persons nor are persons bodies. It is persons – not their bodies – who act and who make choices and have obligations and rights.

According to the report: 'The use of various criteria to define personhood and establish the point at which an embryo or fetus becomes a person is arbitrary and subjective.' (*Church of Scotland*, 1996, p. 56) This claim, I would suggest, embodies a category error. It is not subjective nor arbitrary to try to establish at what point an immature body becomes a person: it is absurd because bodies – no matter how mature they are – are not and never can become persons. I suspect that is it even false to say that an embryo contains within its genetic code all that is needed to become a mature human body. It might contain all the genetic material which it ever will contain and all the genetic material that is required but immature bodies require more than genetic material in order to become mature human bodies. (4)

Even if a human embryo contains the genetic components that are necessary to turn it into a mature human body, this is not a reason for treating an embryo as if it already were a mature human body. B) is false. We should treat things as what they are rather than what they were or will be. My body, like your body, has the potential to become a corpse. It might not become a corpse: it might be blown to smithereens or saved from corruption by the Second Coming. It is a potential corpse but this is not a reason for treating my body or your body as if they already were corpses.

Persons, Genes and Conceptuses

The importance given to 'genes' and to physicality, particularly in a document which has a religious background, is startling. Even if there is a genetic continuity between embryos and the adult bodies of human beings, it does not follow that there are no ethical or theological distinctions between embryos and adult human beings or that differences of treatment of them cannot be ethically justified.

The suggestion is made in the report that: '... the worth of the embryo lies in the fact that it is created in God's image, is genetically complete, and is as much the object of God's concern as the fetus, the child, or the adult...'. (*Church of Scotland*, 1996, p. 59)

Re-reading *Genesis*, I cannot find the claim that embryos – whether or not human ones – were created in God's image. When it is written that humankind – as opposed to the non-human animals – was created in God's image, I do not think that the reference is to our carnality but to some other unspecified feature or features. I adhere to the view that our freedom of the will and our capacity to choose to do good or to do evil is what makes us like God and unlike other animals. (5) To suggest that God is equally concerned with embryos and mature human bodies because both have an equal allowance of genetic material seems to imply that God's love is for genes rather than people. Such a notion seems very odd and disturbing.

According to the report:

'It can further be argued that if we feel unable to affirm that every conceptus is a person, *Psalm* 139 makes it clear that in some cases at least there is a continuity of identity from conceptus to adult'. (*Church of Scotland*, 1996, p. 59)

Now, a 'conceptus' is a fertilised egg. I most certainly am not able to affirm that an egg, whether fertilised or not is a person! It might or might not become the body of one. *Psalm* 139 gives no support at all to the views on embryology and on public policy as suggested in the Church of Scotland's report. What it is says in *Psalm* 139 (verses 15 and 16) is, in the words of King James's Authorised Version:

'15 My substance was not hid from thee, when I was made in secret, and curiously wrought in the lowest parts of the earth.

16 Thine eyes did see my substance, yet being unperfect; and in thy book all my members were written, which in continuation were fashioned, when as yet there was none of them'.

This does not establish the point at all. God is all-knowing and all-seeing. God knows and sees now, before it has been made what, for instance, the new *Ford Fiesta* will look like no less than he knew David before his birth, before, indeed, his conception. What follows from that? It does not follow that eggs are persons. It does not follow that research on *Ford Fiestas* or on human embryos should be illegal.

The report, in similar vein also says:

'Despite natural wastage and the fact that a high proportion of ova do not survive and mature, from a biblical point of view human life begins at conception, at which point the human embryo is genetically complete. The Psalmist traces his identity from adulthood back to his conception (*Psalm* 139). Jeremiah speaks of the fact that even before he was formed in his mother's womb, God had chosen him to be a prophet (*Jeremiah* 1:5)' (*Church of Scotland*, 1996, p. 61)

To say that human life begins at conception is not the same as saying that a person begins as conception or that personal identity starts at conception. Indeed, the point of the verses already quoted from *Psalm* 139 as well as *Jeremiah* 1:5 seems to be quite opposite to the view of the Church of Scotland that personhood starts at conception. *Jeremiah* 1:5 is, again quoting from the Authorised Version, as follows: 'Before I formed thee in the belly I knew thee: and before thou camest forth out of the womb I sanctified thee and I ordained thee a prophet unto the nations'. This seems to me to support my own view that persons and their bodies are distinct rather than the view expressed in the report that persons begin at conception (and end at death?). I think that persons rather than their bodies are moral agents and are the bearers of moral rights. Persons need not have currently existing human bodies in order to have rights. For instance, Donald Dewer the person still has moral rights even although he no longer has a living human body. He has, for instance, the right not to be slandered and, correspondingly, we have a duty not to slander him. Similarly, we have duties towards the persons whose bodies might in future years walk on this planet. I think that those people currently have rights even although they do not currently have live human bodies or even the embryos of them. (See McLachlan, 2002a)

Particular human bodies have a particular physical origination at their conception: it is true but not particularly biblical or significant to say this. That human life begins at conception is not, for all that is shown in the report, a particularly 'biblical' point of view: nor is it at all clear what is being claimed when it is said that human life – as opposed to what? – begins at conception. For neither Christ, Adam nor Eve did human life begin at conception. Consider clones. If someone were born whose body was cloned from another's body, then that person would be due as much moral respect as any other person. Yet, for such a person, human life would not have begun at conception: there would have been no conception.

The Church of Scotland and Bio-ethics Since 1996

Pre-conceived Ideas was published in 1996 under the auspices of the Board of Social Responsibility. Since then, with Donald Bruce as its Director, the Church of Scotland's 'Society, Religion and Technology Project' (S.R.T.) of the Board of National Mission has taken over as the Church of Scotland's most vocal outlet for its accredited views on bio-ethics. It has been particularly vociferous in relation to human cloning, which it abhors. The S.R.T. has been very active politically with highly effective lobbying. It is favourable to the *Report on the Ethical Implications of Biotechnology*, produced by the Advisers to the President of the European Commission, a report which it seems possibly to have influenced. Its press and other media relations and output are highly sophisticated. (6)

The Church of Scotland, the World, the European Union and Cloning

According to the Church of Scotland, the cloning of human beings is unethical and it should be a criminal offence not only in the UK but everywhere in the world. (7) The General Assembly of the Church of Scotland, on the 22nd of May 1997 passed the motion that it would: 'Reaffirm their belief in the basic dignity and uniqueness of each human being under God' and: 'Express the strongest possible opposition to the cloning of human beings and urge Her Majesty's Government to press for a comprehensive international treaty to ban it worldwide'. (8)

It is worth relating the Church's position to the prevailing views in the European Union. For instance the preamble of the resolution on cloning, which was passed by the European parliament on March 13, 1997 is as follows:

'... the cloning of human beings... cannot under any circumstances be justified or tolerated by any society, because it is a serious violation of fundamental human rights and is contrary to the principle of equality of human beings as it permits a eugenic and racist selection of the human race, it offends against human dignity.... [Furthermore, it is the case that] each individual has a right to his or her own genetic identity and that human cloning is, and must continue to be, prohibited'. (9)

In their *Report on the Ethical Implications of Biotechnology*, the Advisers to the President of the European Commission said of reproductive human cloning that: 'Considerations of instrumentalization and eugenics render any such acts ethically unacceptable. In addition, since these techniques entail increased potential risks, safety considerations constitute another ethical objection'. (Advisers, 1997, p. 352)

Harris on Cloning

Harris says of the preamble to the resolution of the European Parliament: 'These statements are ... thin on argument and *rationale*; they appear to have been plucked from the air to justify an instant reaction. There are vague references to "human rights" or "basic principles" with little or no attempt to explain what those principles are, or to indicate how they might apply to cloning'. (Harris, 1997, p. 335)

The case put in the preamble and in the Advisers' report is sketchy and crude. For instance, consider the reference to 'racism' and 'eugenics'. These terms are used more as abusive slogans for attacking cloning than as conceptual tools for analysing it. One might practice 'eugenics' and 'racist selection' by means of normal sexual intercourse no less than by cloning. If one chooses to have sexual intercourse only with one's wife, then one genetically determines and controls the racial origins of any resultant children no less than if one has children through the cloning of one's body. Let us not legislate concerning the motives of people for having children, however they have them. It is worth noting that the Church of Scotland does not, as far as I am aware, promote this particular 'anti-racist' argument.

It is potentially confusing to talk about the cloning of human beings. In this context, distinctions can usefully be made between: persons and their bodies; persons and their minds; persons and their personalities; and, some people would say, persons and their souls. Insofar as cloning might be possible in relation to human beings, it is their bodies and only their bodies that are clonable.

Human cloned bodies would be – and in the case of natural identical twinned bodies actually are – bodies which share the same genetic make-up. If two or more people have bodies with the same genetic make-up, then the persons who have these bodies are – just as much as any other persons – unique persons, if persons are unique. They are, for instance, responsible for their own actions no less than any other persons are. As Harris says:

'Cloning does not produce identical copies of the same individual person. It can only produce identical copies of the same genotype. Our experience of identical twins demonstrates that each is a separate individual with his or her own character, preferences and so on. Although there is some evidence of striking similarities with respect to these factors in twins, there is no question but that each twin is a distinct individual, as independent and as free as anyone else.... We do no feel apprehensive when natural twins are born, why should we when twins are deliberately created?'. (Harris, 1997, p. 353)

Harris suggests that we should not feel apprehensive and, more importantly, that no justification has been given for making human cloning illegal. (10) The pronouncements of the Church of Scotland and of Donald Bruce provide, as we shall see, no such justification.

Ethics, Law, Wisdom and Risk

There are various actions that it would be inappropriate to make illegal – adultery, for instance, and fornication – even if they are ethically unacceptable. The relevant questions here are: is it ethically acceptable to clone human bodies?; whether or not it is ethically acceptable to do so, should it be legal to clone human bodies? I think that, in both cases, the appropriate answer is: yes. It is ethically acceptable to clone human bodies and to do so should be legal. Whether, in any particular circumstances, it would be wise to clone a human body is another question altogether. It would be unwise to try to make unwisdom a criminal offence.

One of the suggested ethical objections to human cloning is that it is risky. In the Church of Scotland's magazine, *Life and Work*, Donald Bruce says it is very unlikely that: '... one would get reproductive human cloning right first time and every time. It would be criminally irresponsible to try. You cannot have a deformed baby "put down" the way you can a suffering lamb'. (Bruce, 2002, p. 21)

I would agree with Bruce that, in the current state of knowledge, it might well be unwise to try to clone a human body. In the present context, it would probably be unethical to do so just as, in many contexts, it might be, for various reasons, unethical for some people to have babies after the normal fashion. However, it does not follow that human cloning should be a crime.

Cloning, just like normal sexual intercourse, might – whether predictably or not – result in the birth of a deformed baby. This is not an argument against either sexual intercourse or cloning in principle as a method of reproduction. Furthermore, since we do not say that it should be a criminal offence to produce by way of normal sexual intercourse – whether or not predictably – a deformed baby there is no obvious reason for saying that it should be a crime to produce a deformed baby by way of cloning. Why should such a thing be criminalised? Who is harmed by the act? The cloned baby? Is it always better not to have been born at all than to have been born deformed? I do not think so. Perhaps it should be a crime to deform a baby that otherwise would have been born un-deformed but that is another matter entirely.

The Uniqueness of Persons and the Supposed Right to Genetic Uniqueness

It says in 'A Supplementary Report to the 1997 General Assembly' from the Society, Religion and Technology Project, Board of National Mission:

'The Church of Scotland has already stated that to clone human beings would be ethically unacceptable as a matter of principle. On principle, to replicate any human technologically is a violation of the basic dignity and uniqueness of each human being made in God's image, of what God has given to that individual to no one else. (11)

I agree – and even if I did not I would be prepared to accept for the sake of the argument – that each of us is created in God's image. However, I cannot see why the cloning of a human body is a violation of anyone's 'basic dignity and uniqueness'. I- the person – have and no one else has, for instance, a unique relationship to the particular body of which the fingers are now typing this sentence on my word processor, to which I also have a unique but less intimate and less profound relationship. Similarly, I have a unique responsibility for my own actions just as you have for yours. People, when they are driving motor vehicles are, uniquely, responsible for some of the movements of the particular vehicles that they are driving. Whether or not the vehicles themselves are physically unique is irrelevant.

Given that twins with the same genetic make-up are natural occurrences (and for other reasons as well), it does not seem to me to be plausible to say that we have a moral right – far less a 'natural' moral right – to unique genetic make-ups. There is much debate about what is meant by a 'moral right' and about what, if anything, our moral rights are grounded upon. The position of the Church of Scotland with regard to the answers to these questions is not made clear. Some people argue that one's rights are related to what one wants or what one needs. For instance, Savulescu writes: 'What constitutes a right is a complex question. On one interpretation, rights protect interests. This implies that a right not to be born would exists if a child had an interest in not being born'. (Savulescu, 2002, p. 65) We do not need to be genetically unique. We can even have – if, say, we needed an organ transplant – an interest in not being genetically unique. Not everyone wants to be genetically unique. Most people, I suspect, don't care whether they are unique or not: they do not think about the matter. Manifestly, those who want to have their bodies cloned do not want genetic uniqueness. Those whose bodies were the result of cloning cannot be presumed to want not to be born.

I take a different approach to rights to the one outlined by Savulescu. In my view, rights are logically related to duties. (12) The rights of one person are either the absences of particular duties as, say, when one has a right (of action) to stand on one's head or else they correspond to the duties of another person or agency (or persons or agencies) as when one has, say, a right (of recipience) to £5 or to life. For instance, I have a natural right to life insofar as it is the duty of all others not to kill me (just as I have a duty not to kill them). I have a (non-natural) moral right to receive £5 if, say, I loaned someone five pounds or if, say, the electricity company over-charged me by £5. On this analysis of rights, one might have rights which one did not need or want. Furthermore, that which we want or need does not automatically become that which others have a moral duty to provide for us and, thereby, that which we have a moral right to receive. For instance, one might want sex; one might even need sex: however, it would not follow that it was necessarily the duty or some person or agency to provide one with sex. A person's wants, interests or needs do not automatically generate particular reflected rights for that person.

On the basis of this duty-based analysis of rights, it is again implausible to claim that people have a right to genetic uniqueness. If you claim to have a right (of recipience) to be genetically unique, it is not clear what you would be claiming as the corresponding duty. It is not clear who or what are being cited as the bearers of the putative duty. Only if all other people have a duty not to have a body with the same genetic make up as mine could it be my natural right that no one else has a body with the same genetic make-up as mine. However, there could be no reason for thinking that all other people have such a duty. If someone had such a body – by chance, by genetic manipulation or whatever – then should we say that he has a duty to cease living in order to preserve my genetic uniqueness? Should I cease living in order to preserve his? The suggestion is implausible.

I was one of twins but my twin miscarried. If we both had the same genetic make-up, how could we both have a right and an equal right to have it uniquely? How could we simultaneously have a duty and an equal duty not to have it? It is not apparent that we could.

Donald Bruce says, when trying to show 'Why the Cloning of Humans is Ethically Unacceptable' that: 'Christians would see this as a violation of the uniqueness of a human life, which God has given to each of us and to no one else'. (13) However, Bruce gives no reason at all for suggesting that it is a tenet of Christianity that God gave each one of us – other, of course, than identical twins – unique gene-sets. The notion seems to me to be a groundless superstition. We do not require to have such unique gene-sets in order to lead unique lives or, rather, to live uniquely similar lives. Each and every human being deserves human dignity but we deserve this dignity whether or not we have non-identical gene-sets. We can be unique as individual persons and have, for instance, unique souls without being uniquely genetically branded. God can identify each and every one of us without recourse to the customization of our flesh.

I do not think that we have a right to bodily uniqueness. However, our bodies might be physically unique whether or not we have a right (of recipience) to such uniqueness. (14) Furthermore, human cloning is not incompatible with bodily uniqueness. The Church of Scotland's representatives seem to be bedazzled and bemused by the very thought of genes. They attach a sort of mystical and misplaced importance to them. (15) Cloned bodies are not necessarily identical bodies. For instance, identical twins do not have identical fingerprints. (16) Bodies are causally affected by factors other than their genes. (17) This is particularly so in the case of cloned bodies since, unlike natural twins, they would develop in different wombs.

The Occurrence of Twins and the Production of Clones

Bruce is right to say that deliberate cloning is not necessarily morally equivalent to the occurrence of natural twins. That which happens should often be distinguished from that which is done even when the outcomes are identical. (18) For instance, it might be a good outcome were, say, an aged and suffering relative to die, but a bad action to kill her. Many people would say that Judas's betrayal of Christ was a bad action – one in breech of Judas's duty of loyalty to his friend and Master – however good and glorious they consider Christ's consequent crucifixion and its aftermath to have been. However, it does not follow that cloning is wrong. If you say people have a duty not to clone human bodies, then you will be asked what the grounds of such a suggested duty are. It cannot be people's natural right to genetic uniqueness since there is no such natural right. By definition, the natural rights of each person are the same as those of all people, including twins. What could the grounds of such a suggested duty be?

According to Donald Bruce:

'The mere existence of "identical" twins cannot be cited to justify the practice of cloning... it is not the genetic identity that is the crucial point but the human act of control, and it is this element of control which provides the fundamental ethical case against human cloning.... Such control by one human over another is incompatible with the ethical notion of human freedom, in the sense that each individual's genetic identity should be inherently unpredictable and unplanned'. (19)

Consider also the following claims made by him in *Life and Work*:

'Cloning is a deliberate act where someone takes the genetic composition of another person and makes a new individual with the same genes. [An] intrinsic ethical objection to human cloning is that no human being should be given such power to predetermine another person's complete genetics.... Our genes remain fixed and unalterable. It is an inappropriate power to give to any human the power to pre-determine them'. (Bruce, 2002, p. 21)

Notice that, *pace* Bruce, the debate is not about what powers people ought to have or ought to be given. Perhaps it would be better if no one had the power to produce cloned bodies. Perhaps, too, it would be better if some people did not have the power to have, in the normal way, children. The relevant questions are, given the some people might have the ability to clone human bodies: would it be necessarily immoral to exercise such power?; should to be illegal to do so? To both questions, the correct answer is, I think: no. Nothing that the Church of Scotland or its representatives say substantiates the contrary positions.

Why should each individual's genetic identity be inherently unpredictable and unplanned? Bruce does not say. If you have sex with and only with your wife then the genetic make-up of any children that you have will be, to an extent, predictable and planned. The genes of your children will be determined by your actions no less than if their bodies were cloned. In both cases, your children will have no more or less choice over what their genes will be. Human freedom is about the capability of persons as persons to choose what their actions will be: it is not about the particular genetic make up of their bodies or about whether their gene-sets were in any sense chosen for them or allocated to them totally randomly.

Christianity and Kantianism

In relation to instrumentality and human cloning, Donald Bruce says on the SRT Project's web-site: 'To replicate any human being technologically is a fundamentally instrumental act towards two unique individuals – the one from whom the clone is taken and the clone itself'. (20)

There is a confusion here between (unique) persons and their (unique or non-unique) bodies. Cloning can certainly be seen as the instrumental use of parts of a human body in order, deliberately, to produce another (genetically identical) body. However, it is not apparent that this instrumental use of genetic material is necessarily the abuse of a person. What person is being abused? Consider the person whose body is the source of the genetic material. Why should we say that this person is being abused and/or exploited? What if permission were given by the person for the procedure? Consider the person whose body the copied genetic material might serve to produce. Why should one say that this person is being ill-treated? It is not credible to say that oblivion would be preferable to life with a non-unique gene-set.

Consider Bruce's argument in conjunction with the following claim from the previously discussed report of the Church of Scotland's Study Group on Human Fertilisation and Embryology:

'At every stage of life a human being must be treated as a person, enjoying a unique status and of supreme value to God. No person can rightly be treated as a means to an end. If we accord to the human embryo the full rights of a person, then all research on human embryos must be morally wrong'. (Church of Scotland, 1996, p. 62)

This is not so much Christianity as a misunderstanding and a misapplication of Kantianism. (See Acton, 1970 and Harris, 1997) People can be rightly treated as means to an end: this is not seriously disputed. That they must not be treated *merely* as that is Kant's contention. To treat a *body* – rather than a person – as an end in itself, even to treat it merely as that can sometimes be an appropriate thing to do. Not all research on human embryos is the wrongful treatment of a person: at least, the arguments of the Church of Scotland's study group do not show that it is. Furthermore, and more importantly, they do that show that – whether or not it is morally wrong – it should be illegal. For instance, suicide might be, as Kant contends, always morally wrong. Whether or not it should always (or ever) be illegal is another matter.

One might, in my view, obey Christ's injunction to love God and love one's neighbour as one's self and support research on human embryos. Persons – not embryos or any other sort of bodies – are our neighbours. Christopher Reeve, the paralysed actor who played the part of Superman, is our neighbour. It is difficult for me to see how I could love him as I love myself and yet seek to thwart research that might help him to walk again.

It says too in the report:

'We believe that everyone is created in the image of God and is called in Christ to manifest that likeness. Each person is loved by God and is of supreme value. As such, each person, irrespective of who he or she is, enjoys equality of dignity and status with every other person before God and must be treated with appropriate respect'. (*Church of Scotland*, 1996, p. 9)

I, as a member of the Church of Scotland, believe too that everyone is created in the image of God and is called in Christ to manifest that likeness. I do not believe that each embryo is created in the image of God. Every person, of course, must be treated with appropriate respect. This is a tautology even if an important one. However, what counts as appropriate respect (as well as what counts as a person) is precisely what is at issue here. I deny that the arguments of the report show that research on human embryos is inconsistent with the respect that it is appropriate to accord to persons.

Conclusion

There is room for much debate about the proper relationship between law and ethics as well as between religion and law and between religion and ethics. (21) Ethics and politics are distinct from each other and are distinct from religion, particularly when that religion is Christianity. Christianity is a religion of salvation: it is not, in any straight-forward sense, a programme for political action or even a code of ethics. Religious, ethical and political positions need to be defended in their own terms even if it turns out – as it sometimes but not invariably does – that there is an affinity between some particular sound religious and sound ethical and/or political positions. For instance, the Church of Scotland is opposed to sins but is not thereby wedded to the view that all sins *qua* sins should be crimes. It is a sin, let us say, to commit adultery, to covet one's neighbour's ass and to fail to honour one's mother and father. It does not follow that these things should be, or that we should strive to make them, crimes. Even if human cloning and research on human embryos were sinful, it does not follow that they should be illegal. The wisdom of making them illegal, particularly in a 'multi-cultural' society, would need to be established in secular terms.

In general, the derivation of ethical and/or political positions from Christianity is problematical. In particular, the views of the Church of Scotland on the ethics and appropriate legal status of human cloning and of research on human embryos cannot readily be shown to follow from an acceptance of Christianity. I would insist that my own views as here expressed are no less Christian than the official Church of Scotland ones are. Of more importance and of more general interest and concern, the arguments of the Church on human cloning and research on embryos are weak ones, whether or not they are particularly congruent with Christianity. In relation to the theology and ethics of cloning, one might simply 'agree to differ' with the Church of Scotland's positions. However, when these views concern the criminal law, they impinge on all of us and, insofar as they are unreasonable, they should be opposed.

*By Hugh V. McLachlan, from *Scottish Affairs*, 2004, No. 46, pp. 110-130

Footnotes

(1) See McLachlan and Swales, 2000, for a related discussion of the position of the Church of Scotland on surrogate motherhood.

(2) The Study Group on Human Fertilisation and Embryology was convened by the Rev. David Easton and the Board of Social Responsibility was convened by the Rev. William Wallace. The report was presented to the General Assembly of the Church of Scotland in 1996 and there was a deliverance passed commending it. The conclusions of the report were all passed as deliverances.

(3) The Warnock Committee (1984) took the view that the pre-implantation embryo has not achieved the same moral or legal status as the fully formed fetus. This view seems to have been accepted by Parliament in the Human Fertilisation and Embryology Act (1990). For a reasonably comprehensive account of the range of the debate, see Green, 2001. See also Fox, 2000 and McLachlan, 2002a and 2002b.

(4) See, for instance, Ridley, 2003 and King, 2003.

(5) See Broadie, 2000, for a brilliant, succinct and fascinating account of – among other central issues in Scottish philosophy – the differences between the philosophies of human action of David Hume and Thomas Reid. It is interesting to note that the views of the Study Group seem more in accord with those

of Hume, the celebrated atheist and mine are more like those of Thomas Reid. Reid, as well as being a better although not a better-known philosopher than Hume was also a Church of Scotland minister.

(6) See, for instance its web-site: (http://dspace.dial.pipex.com/srtscot/gmanimal.htm) It has produced reports for the General Assembly and a book: *Engineering Genesis*, Bruce and Bruce, 1998.

(7) In the past when the Church of Scotland lobbied successfully to have, for instance witchcraft, bestiality and adultery made crimes – and capital crimes at that – it stopped short of world-wide bans. See Maxwell-Stuart, 2001, pp. 35-45.

(8) See: http://dspace.dial.pipex.com/srtscot/ga97clon.htm. See also 'Cloning Animals and Humans', Supplementary Reports to the Church of Scotland's General Assembly, May 1997, p. 36/22, and Board of National Mission deliverances 35 and 36, p. 16.

(9) The European Parliament. The motion is dated March 11 1997.

(10) See also Harris, 1998 and McLachlan, 2002a. For another expression of a view different from Harris's and mine, see Gogarty, 2003.

(11) See: http://dspace.dial.pipex.com/srtscot/ga97clon.htm.

(12) On the relationship between rights and duties see Raphael, 1971, p. 68 and O'Neill, 2002, pp. 78-82. See also: McLachlan, 1973; 1997a: and 1998. See also Freeden, 1991 and Campbell *et al.*, 1986.

(13) See: http://dspace.dial.pipex.com/srtscot/clonhum2.htm.

(14) We have, of course, a right of action to genetic uniqueness: we are not dutibound not to be genetically unique.

(15) Bodies and clones of that body should not be thought of as being like, say, reading lists and photocopies of reading lists. According to Ridley, it is also a mistake to regard genes as being like the blue-prints of a body: genes, he suggests are more like recipes. Dishes made from the same recipe are not always identical. See Ridley, 2003.

(16) I have argued elsewhere that even if people do have identical finger-prints, it is not known nor it is knowable either *a priori* or *a posteriori* that they do. It is mere superstition to say that each person must have a unique set of finger-prints (or, by the same reasoning, a unique set of genes or any other physical feature or arrangement of features). See McLachlan, 1995.

(17) Lederberg makes the very interesting point that we must

look beyond the human genome as the cause of our bodily states, features and conditions since: '... much of the biological composition of our bodies consists of genomes other than the human. Multitudes of bacteria and viruses occupy our skin, our mucous membranes and our intestinal tract'. (Lederberg, 2003, p. 15). He goes on to say that: 'It would thus broaden our philosophical horizons if we thought of a human as more than an organism. It is a super-organism with an extended genome that includes not only its own cells, but also the fluctuating microbial genome set of bacteria and viruses which share that body space'. (2003, p. 15)

(18) See McLachlan and Swales, 1999.

(19) See: http://dspace.dial.pipex.com/srtscot/clonhum2.htm.

(20) See: http://dspace.dial.pipex.com/srtscot/clonhum2.htm.

(21) See, for instance, McHale and Fox with Murphy, 1991, chapter 2; Brazier, 1992, chapters 2 and 22; and McLachlan, 1997b. Religious commandments – think, for instance, of the famous Ten – are what they are: commandments. They are not ethical principles. They are not assertions of what is the case: they are neither true nor false. (See McLachlan, 1979) 'Keep off the grass', for instance, is neither true nor false. Commands are, rather, wise or un-wise and authoritative or non-authoritative. 'Thou shalt not' does not mean the same as 'It is morally wrong to...'.

References

Acton, H.B., 1970, *Kant's Moral Philosophy*, Macmillan, London.

Advisers to the President of the European Commission on the Ethical Implications of Biotechnology, 1997, 'Ethical Aspects of Cloning Techniques', *Journal of Medical Ethics*, Vol. 23, No. 6, pp. 349-352

Brazier, M., 1992, *Medicine, Patients and the Law*, Penguin Books.

Broadie, Alexander, 2000, *Why Scottish Philosophy Matters*, The Saltire Society, Edinburgh.

Bruce, Donald 2001, 'Human Embryonic Cloning', *Human Reproduction and Genetic Ethics*, Vol. 7, No. 1, pp. 3-7.

Bruce, Donald 2002, 'Running on the Spot: The ethics of the new technologies', *Life and Work*, April, pp. 19-21.

Bruce, D. and Bruce. A (editors), 1998, *Engineering Genesis*, Earthscan, London.

Campbell, T. *et al.* (eds), 1986, *Human Rights: From Rhetoric to Reality*, Oxford, Blackwell.

Church of Scotland, (1996), *Pre-conceived Ideas: A Christian Perspective of IVF and Embryology*, Church of Scotland, Study Group on Human Fertilisation and Embryology, St. Andrews Press, Edinburgh.
Fox, Marie, 2000, 'Pre-persons, Commodities or Cyborgs? The Legal Construction and Representation of the Embryo', *Health Care Analysis*, Vol. 8, pp. 171-181.
Freeden, M., 1991, *Rights*, Milton Keynes, Open University.
Gogarty, B., 2003, 'What exactly is a copy? And why it matters when trying to ban reproductive cloning in Australia', *Journal of Medical Ethics*, vol. 29, pp. 84-89.
Green, R.M., 2001, *The Human Embryo Research Debates: Bioethics in the Vortex of Controversy*, Oxford University Press.
Harris, John, 1997, '"Goodbye Dolly?" The Ethics of Human Cloning', *Journal of Medical Ethics*, Vol. 23, No. 6, pp. 353360.
Harris, John, 1998, *Clones, Genes and Immortality: Ethics and the Genetic Revolution*, Oxford University Press, Oxford.
King, David (2003), 'Just How Complex is Genetics Really?', *Human Reproduction and Genetic Ethics*, Vol. 9, No. 1, pp. 13-15.
Lederberg, Joshua, 2003, 'Learning from our complex relationship with bugs', *The Herald*, April 26, p. 15.
McHale, J. and Fox M. with Murhpy, J., 1991, *Health Care Law: Text and Materials*, London, Sweet and Maxwell.
McLachlan, Hugh V., 1973, 'The Right to Work', *Contemporary Review*, June, pp. 307-311.
McLachlan, Hugh V., 1979, 'The Is/Ought Question: A Needless Controversy', *Journal of the British Society for Phenomenology*, Vol. 10, No. 2, pp. 134-137.
McLachlan, Hugh V., 1995, 'No Two Sets Exactly the Same? Applying Philosophy to the Theory of Fingerprints', *The Philosopher*, Vol. 83, No. 2, pp. 12-18.
McLachlan, Hugh V., 1997a, 'Bodies, Rights and Abortion', *Journal of Medical Ethics*, Vol. 23, No. 3, pp. 176-180.
McLachlan, Hugh V., 1997b, 'Defending Commercial Surrogate Motherhood Against Van Nierkerk and Van Zyl', *Journal of Medical Ethics*, Vol. 23, No. 6, pp. 344-348.
McLachlan, Hugh V., 1998, 'Justice, Rights and Health Care: A Discussion of the Report of the Commission on Social Justice', *International Journal of Sociology and Social Policy*, Vol. 18, Nos. 11/12, pp. 65-84.

McLachlan, Hugh V., 2002a, 'Bodies, Persons and Research on Human Embryos', *Human Reproduction and Genetic Ethics*, Vol. 8, No. 1.
McLachlan, Hugh V., 2002b, 'Persons and Their Bodies: How We Should Think About Human Embryos', *Health Care Analysis*, Vol. 10, No. 2, pp. 155-164.
McLachlan, Hugh V. and Swales, J. Kim, 1999, 'A Drunk Driver, A Sober Pedestrian and the Allocation of Tragically Scarce and Indivisible Emergency Hospital Treatment', *Health Care Analysis*, Vol. 7, No. 1, pp. 5-21.
McLachlan, Hugh V. and Swales, J. Kim, 2000, 'Scotland, the Church and Surrogate Motherhood', *Scottish Affairs*, No. 32, Summer, pp. 110-123.
Maxwell-Stuart, P.G., 2001, *Satan's Conspiracy: Magic and Witchcraft in Sixteenth-Century Scotland*, Tuckwell Press, East Linton.
O'Neill, Onora, 2002, *Autonomy and Trust in Bioethics*, Cambridge, Cambridge University Press, pp. 78-82.
Raphael, D.D., 1971, *Problems of Political Philosophy*, London, Macmillan, p. 68.
Ridley, Matt, 2003, *Nature Via Nurture: Genes, Experience and What Makes us Human*, London, Fourth Estate.
Savulescu, J., 2002, 'Is there a "right not to be born?": Reproductive decision making, options and the right to information', *Journal of Medical Ethics*, Vol. 28, pp. 65-67.

Chapter Seven

Unique Persons and the Replicable Gene-sets of their Reproducible Bodies: A Defence of Human Cloning*

Introduction

The assertion that human reproductive cloning should become a criminal offence where it is not already prohibited is claimed by those who make it to be an extraordinarily popular one. Perhaps it is amongst the present general public. There is a minor public outcry whenever the claim is made that someone has succeeded in producing or is even attempting to produce what is referred to as 'a cloned human being'. However, amongst academic commentators, the case against such cloning in principle has by no means gained universal, unqualified support. Problems with the arguments put forward in support of the anti-cloning position have frequently been pointed out [1] The debate about human reproductive cloning should not be thought of as having been rationally concluded. It is not over yet. In the general public arena, it has scarcely begun. I have no hopes or expectations of settling all the issues here but I do intend to show the inadequacy of the typical attacks on human reproductive cloning. In this respect, the case referred to by Gogarty shall be cited as an example [2].

Gogarty says of human reproductive cloning: '... there is a widespread community consensus that the activity should be prohibited' [3]. It is not illegal in all countries. Gogarty wishes that it were and advocates the universal adoption of the UK legislation whereby, in terms of the Human Reproductive Cloning Act (2001): 'A person who places in a woman a human embryo which has been created otherwise than by fertilisation is guilty of an offence'. He gives a brief and uncritical account of a cluster of arguments which opponents of human cloning who – like Gogarty himself – want it to be illegal commonly employ in their attack of it. He says:

'... this is a far from comprehensive list of objections to human cloning. It is, however, sufficient to note that these reflect a variety of views held by various sectors of the community. In a world divided by ethical, political and social differences such a near universal consensus is rare' [4].

In this paper, the validity and force of the arguments on Gogarty's list shall be examined. The conclusion is reached that, contrary to what Gogarty suggests, human cloning should not be a crime. As a prelude to that examination, some remarks on the nature of cloning and on the alleged consensus of opinion against it will be made.

The nature of human cloning

Gogarty says:

'For the purposes of this paper, the term [i.e. 'reproductive cloning'] is taken to mean any embryo produced by a process other than fertilisation, which is implanted into a human body, with the intention of replicating an existing individual, alive or dead' [5].

According to Gogarty:

'The idea of producing children that are exact replicas of living (or deceased) people has received near unanimous condemnation by the world community. The UNESCO Declaration on the Human Genome and Human Rights 1997 states that "practices such as reproductive cloning of human beings shall not be permitted". The document has been signed by 186 nations, reflecting international consensus on many ethical issues in the application of biotechnology to humans' [3].

Objections to the replication of people as people – if such a notion is an intelligible one – are beside the point here. Gogarty's analysis of what human cloning means is misconceived. Human cloning is not about the replication of people. Persons *have*, for instance, bodies, minds and personalities. However, persons *are not* bodies, nor minds, nor personalities. In so far as cloning involves replication, it is the replication of gene-sets. Persons are never replicated. Human cloning is not even the replication of bodies since cloned bodies cannot be expected to be identical any more than so-called 'identical twins' are identical. Such twins are physically very similar but they are not identical. That they do not have identical fingerprints is only one of the physical differences between them [6]. They seem more physically similar than they actually are because of the vagaries and imperfections of our organs of perception particularly of our sight and our fixation with faces. The bodies of 'identical twins' are not like two photocopies of the same document. They are not replicas. Bodies are affected by numerous and various causal factors and not merely by their genes [7].

Ridley argues that it is a commonly made mistake to regard genes as being like the blue-prints of a body: genes, he suggests are more like recipes. He points out that dishes made from the same recipe are not always identical [8]. According to Lederberg, there is a danger of over-emphasising the importance of our own genomes in relation to the causes of our bodily states, features and conditions. It is his contention that: '... much of the biological composition of our bodies consists of genomes other than the human. Multitudes of bacteria and viruses occupy our skin, our mucous membranes and our intestinal tract' [9]. He claims: 'It would thus broaden our philosophical horizons if we thought of a human [body] as more than an organism. It is a super-organism with an extended genome that includes not only its own cells, but also the fluctuating microbial genome set of bacteria and viruses which share that body space' [9].

Human cloning is not the production of children who are the exact replicas of living or deceased people. It is a misunderstanding (or a series of misunderstandings) to suppose that it is. It is not even the reproduction of identical bodies. Harris writes:

'Cloning does not produce identical copies of the same individual person. It can only produce identical copies of the same genotype.... Artificial clones do not raise any difficulties not raised by the phenomenon of "natural" twins. We do not feel apprehensive when natural twins are born, why should we when twins are deliberately created?' [10].

Twins – however similar their bodies might be – are individual persons just like any one else. They might but might not have similar personalities, tastes, interests, *etc.*

The Tyranny of Actual and Alleged Majorities

I am not convinced that there really is the level of opposition to human cloning that Gograty claims. He has not shown that it amounts to 'a near universal consensus'. He says that 186 countries have signed a particular declaration but he does not tell us how many countries there are in the world: how many countries have not signed it? One can infer from what he says about his own country of Australia – although he does not actually point this out himself – that, of its six federal states, cloning is illegal in only three of them. It would be naive to imagine that governments always agree with all the treaties that they sign. Furthermore, if Mr. Blair and Mr. Bush, on behalf of the UK and the USA, sign a particular treaty, it does not follow that everyone in both of these countries agrees with the treaty. It does not even follow that a majority of people in these countries agrees with the text. People can, in any case, change their minds.

The significance of the claimed popularity of the opposition to cloning is not clear. If a particular law is not a justifiable law, it will not become one merely because a majority of people within a particular jurisdiction want it to be enacted. As J.S. Mill argues, the tyranny of the majority is not less tyrannical and as such no more justified than the tyranny of the minority [11]. Even if every one in the world wanted human cloning to be a criminal offence, this, in my view, would not be a sufficient justification for making it a crime. Restrictions on the freedom of people to perform specified actions and, more particularly, the threat and actuality of punishment when they do perform them always requires to be morally justifiable. Sufficient reason for moral justification must be presentable and the fact that some or all people want the restriction, the punishment and the threat of it to be imposed is not sufficient reason: it is no moral reason at all. It might, in some jurisdictions at least, suffice to make the law legally legitimate but legal and moral legitimacy are different things.

Suppose that most people in a particular jurisdiction and/or in the world wanted homosexual acts to be illegal. Would this desire be in itself a moral justification for criminalising homosexual acts? I do not think so. Even if every person in a jurisdiction and/or in the world at any particular time wanted homosexual acts to be illegal, I do not think that this would be a justification for making such acts illegal. According to J.S. Mill, it is justifiable to make an action illegal only if – but not always if – the action harms some one other than the actor. I am not sure that I would want to be as specific as Mill or to offer such a general answer to the question of why and when legislation is justifiable [12]. There might be various sorts of justifications for different sorts of laws in different contexts and circumstances. However, I think that Mill is correct in suggesting that, whereas there is no requirement to justify the absence of particular criminal laws, the onus is always on those who want to outlaw particular activities to justify the prohibition. The mere desire for the prohibition (however popular and however strongly felt) does not constitute nor even count towards a justification.

The making of human cloning a criminal offence

Gogarty's list of 'objections to human cloning' comes under six headings: risk; diversity; lack of need; human dignity; autonomy; and individuality. Each argument – whether or not it identifies a reasonable objection to particular instances of human cloning – is defective when considered as a grounds for making the procedure of human cloning a criminal offence. After all, in general, objections can sometimes reasonably be made to various activities even if they do not necessarily constitute grounds for making the activity a crime. For instance, there might be reasonable objections – including ethical ones – to voting for one or more of the following political parties (in Scotland) in some circumstances and contexts: the British National Party; the Scottish National Party; the Scottish Socialist Party; the Labour Party. It does not follow that it would be reasonable to make any of these actions crimes. Similarly, there can be objections – including ethical ones – to some instances of human sexual reproduction although it would not be reasonable to make either human sexual reproduction as such nor the particular instances of it a crime.

Consider Gogarty's arguments in turn.

Risk

One reads: 'The most common objection to cloning humans is that the current technology is unsafe' [3]. In all likelihood, as Gogarty indicates, there would be few live births as a result of human cloning at present and those babies that were born would: '... have a high chance of dying from heart and blood vessel problems, malformed arteries, diabetes, immune system deficiencies, and physical deformities' [3].

I share this objection to cloning in the sense that I agree that it would be unwise to clone human beings at present and, probably, unethical to do so. However, the argument from 'risk' does not constitute firm grounds for making human cloning a criminal offence. Normal sexual human reproduction can be risky. Indeed, in certain instances of normal sexual procreation, the chances that a baby will be malformed are very high. However, such instances of sexual intercourse are not crimes. I do not think that they should be crimes. However, if the risk involved were sufficient grounds for making human cloning a crime, it would be sufficient grounds for making such normal intercourse a crime. I think that neither human cloning nor sexual intercourse with known risk should be, on the grounds of such risk, illegal.

Lack of need

This leads to the supposed argument against human cloning in terms of 'lack of need'. Gogarty writes: 'An objection commonly raised by scientists, but which also verges on the ethical, is that there is little or no scientific or medical justification for cloning... motives for human cloning are based on increasing personal notoriety rather than the greater good'[4].

It would be foolish to legislate with regard to people's motives for having children whatever reproductive technique – whether natural or non-natural – they choose to use. With normal sexual intercourse, people have children for all sorts of motives. People do not normally have children 'for the greater good'. I would be very suspicious of people who had children for such a motive although I would not want to make their actions in having them criminal offences. If people have children in order to increase their personal notoriety and use the method of normal sexual intercourse then their actions are not criminal. If it should be a crime to have a cloned baby in order to increase one's personal notoriety, then it should be a crime to have a baby for that reason whatever technique one chooses to use.

It is curious to cite lack of need as grounds for making an action illegal. It can hardly be suggested as a serious principle that actions should be crimes unless the actions can be shown to be necessary. Of any particular instance of normal reproductive sexual intercourse, one might truly say that it was not scientifically nor medically necessary. But lack of need is not the same as lack of a required justification. Legality does not require a justification. The onus, rather, is on those who want to outlaw actions to justify the prohibition.

Human dignity

Gogarty indicates that a commonly expressed ethical objection to human cloning – as made, for instance, in declarations of so-called 'human rights' by the Council of Europe and UNESCO – is that it is 'contrary to human dignity'. He notes that:

'The Anglican diocese of Melbourne submitted to the Andrews committee that cloning was instrumental in nature because it: "bring[s] a person into existence for reasons outside the person themselves ... to clone is to exercise unprecedented control over the genetic dimension of another individual...'[4].

Gogarty continues: 'Indeed, this element of control over the genetic make up of successive generations is evocative of concepts of eugenics which were rejected by the world community after the second world war'[4].

Normal sexual intercourse, no less than human cloning brings human beings into existence 'for reasons outside the person[s] themselves'. Normal sexual intercourse no less than human cloning causes the genetic make up of consequent babies. To clone is not necessarily to *control* genetic make-up. Control, in any case, is not necessarily morally wrong. Even if it were, it does not follow that it should be illegal. One might control the genetic make up of one's children by deliberately having sexual intercourse only with particular people and/or only with what one considered to be particular sorts of people. This should also be a criminal offence if cloning is criminalised on the grounds that it could be used for 'eugenic' reasons.

Some people reject particular beliefs and practices – such as, for instance, 'eugenics' – because they associate them with Adolf Hitler and the Nazis. On that basis, one should reject, for instance, vegetarianism and public works schemes for combating unemployment. True ideas do not become false merely because Hitler believed them nor do practices become evil merely because the Nazis performed them. What, if it is wrong, is immoral with eugenics? If cloning should be illegal, why should it be illegal? These questions cannot be dismissed by saying that the 'world community' – whatever such a community might be – rejects concepts of 'eugenics'.

Diversity

Gogarty's argument under the heading of 'diversity' is, as putative grounds for making human cloning a crime, off target. He says:

'Cloning presents, albeit if taken to the extreme, a departure from human diversity. By undertaking asexual reproduction, the gene pool will be narrowed and humanity's ability to overcome disease will be constrained. Cloning represents what some see as a "slippery slope" towards unwarranted and unmanaged interference with evolutionary development'[4].

Cloning as such will not decrease genetic diversity. Indeed, from the point of view of genetic diversity, it would be better that I were succeeded by a clone than that I were childless. Failure to produce children by sexual reproduction might count towards threatening genetic diversity but to suggest that it should be – on that account (or on any other account) – a criminal offence to be wilfully childless is an absurdity.

Autonomy

Gogarty writes:

'Opponents of cloning claim that the free will and autonomy of a clone would be severely impacted upon either intentionally of by virtue of continuing comparisons with their genetic parent. The instinct to direct that child's development, they argue, would be strong. Even where there was no substantial pressure to mirror the achievements of the clonal parent, the clone would live in the shadow if its predecessor'[4].

If this is what the opponents of cloning believe, then we might remind them that they need not have clones of their own. However, what they believe is no reason for criminalising the activity. It might be tough to be a clone, but this is no reason for making human cloning a criminal offence. It is tough to be a human being of any sort, or it can be: it is still, I would suggest, better to have been born than not to exist, in all or virtually all instances. One is hardly doing a clone a favour by sparing him the hardships of life by denying him life. Even if it turns out that a particular life was not worth *living*, it might still have been worth *having* for the sake of its potential.

Should it be a crime, for example, for kings, prime ministers, pop stars and philosophical geniuses to have children because of the pressures that their fame will cause for their children? One cannot reasonably think so. In any case, there is no reason for believing that the pressure on cloned children would be, in general, any greater than that on other children of famous or non-famous parents. Sometimes, unsuccessful and non-famous parents are particularly anxious that their children should shine prominently, thereby causing their offspring a lot of stress and embarrassment.

Individuality

Gogarty presents a pot-pourri of interesting but unconvincing claims when he says:

'Cloning is said to breach a fundamental right to individuality. By allowing cloning, humanity would be foregoing the intrinsic knowledge that each person is new and unique, not predetermined, prejudged, or prejudiced by what has gone before or after each person. Uniqueness of identity and individuality are some of the most deeply felt and inherent signifiers of self. Just as great artwork would lose its value in identical reproductions, so human beings can be said to lose their intrinsic inimitability in reproductions of themselves'[4].

Human cloning is not the identical reproduction of human beings. Even if it were, Gogarty's argument is unconvincing. Persons whose bodies are cloned from someone else's body are no more or less than other people free to choose to do particular things. They are no more nor less likely than other people to be influenced by what is expected of them.

Some – although not all – individuals might have a very strong feeling regarding their own uniqueness: such feelings do not indicate the presence of, nor generate the existence of, moral rights to uniqueness.

Works of art may have both aesthetic value and economic value. The former, unlike the latter, is not affected by reproduction. Both senses of 'value' are different from the inherent moral worth of individual persons. For instance, if Leonardo Da Vinci had painted ten copies of the Mona Lisa and the copies were absolutely identical then all ten copies would have the same inherent aesthetic worth. Whether they would all sell for the same sum of money as a unique Mona Lisa is another matter.

There are important respects in which we have individuality and uniqueness (whether or not we have a *right* to them). Human cloning is no threat to such individuality and uniqueness. Persons as persons are unique individuals. Whether or not their bodies, their personality traits, their minds, their gene-sets or any other such characteristics are individual and/or unique is quite beside the point. Persons have, for instance, a unique relationship with their own bodies, minds and so forth. Persons are the unique bearers of particular rights and duties. Individual persons are uniquely responsible and blameworthy or praiseworthy for particular actions of their own. For example, if I steal a pot of jam from a supermarket or – more likely, I hope – rescue a child from a blazing building, then I – and only I – should be punished or praised as the unique and individual author of the particular action. The replication of gene-sets and the question of the uniqueness of physical attributes and of combinations of them are totally irrelevant. Consider an analogy. Even if every motorcar were identical, each driver would be an individual driver and would have a unique, particular responsibility for the manoeuvres of the vehicle which he drives.

Conclusion

Although I am a defender of, I do not consider myself to be an advocate of human reproductive cloning. For instance, I am not trying to hasten its occurrence. I do not consider it important whether or not it ever occurs. I would not be displeased were it never to occur. However, in relation to public policy as in private life, it is often important to stress not merely what is done but also how and why what is done is done. For a variety of reasons, it is, in general, important that we do not accept bad arguments as the basis for public policy. For instance, we should oppose weak arguments because acceptance of them, even tacit or apparent acceptance, debases the currency of public debate. Since people often think – misguidedly, perhaps – that consistency is a great virtue in legal systems, bad and unjustified legislation begets further bad, unjustified legislation. In addition, it is important that we do not accept these particularly deficient anti-cloning arguments. They are based on a misunderstanding of what human cloning is. It is insulting and antithetical to human dignity to suggest that the (supposed) physical uniqueness of their bodies is a condition of the inherent moral worth of individual people.

The arguments suggested by Gogarty in support of the criminalisation of human cloning are defective. Of these arguments, he says: '... this is a far from comprehensive list of objections to cloning'[4]. This is a surprising remark since the arguments cited by him are the ones those who declare that human cloning should be a crime are in the habit of making. [13]. Why would such people use these weak arguments if better ones were available [14]? It is possible that there are other good arguments for making human reproductive cloning illegal that have not yet been made public. Unless they are forthcoming, human reproductive cloning should be legalised where it has been made a crime and remain legal where it is legal.

*By Hugh V McLachlan, from *Human Reproduction and Genetic Ethics*, 2005, Vol. 11, No. 2, pp. 43-48.

Footnotes and References

(1) In particular, see Caulfield, T. (2003) 'Human Cloning Laws, Human Dignity and the Poverty of the Policy Making Dialogue' *BMC Medical Ethics*, 4:3 (Open Access, On-line, Biomed Central journal available at http://www.biomedcentral.com/1472-6939/4/3 and Harris, J. (1997) '"Goodbye Dolly?" The Ethics of Human Cloning', *Journal of Medical Ethics*, 23, pp. 353-360.

See also, for instance: Beyleverd D. and Brownsword R. (1998) 'Human Dignity, Human Rights and Human Genes', *The Modern Law Review*, 1998, 61, pp. 661-681; Buchanan, A., Brock D., Daniels N., Wikler D. (2000) *From Chance to Choice: Genetics and Justice*. Cambridge, Cambridge University Press; Harris, J. (1999) 'Clones, Genes and Human Rights' in J Burley, editor, *The Genetic Revolution and Human Rights*, Oxford, Oxford University Press pp. 61-94; McLachlan, H.V. (2004) 'Human Embryos, Clones and Public Policy: A Critique of The Church of Scotland's Views', *Scottish Affairs*, 46, Winter; Malby, S. (2002) 'Human Dignity and Human Reproductive Cloning' *Health and Human Rights*, 6, pp. 103-135; Robertson J. (1994) 'The Question of Human Cloning',

Hastings Center Report, 24, pp. 6-14; Robertson J. (1998) 'Liberty, Identity and Human Cloning', *Texas Law Review*, 76, pp. 1371-1456; Pattison S. (2002) 'Reproductive Cloning: Can Cloning Harm the Clone?', *Medical Law Review*, 10 pp. 295-307; Rovane C. (2002) 'Genetics and Personal Identity' in *A Companion to Genetic Ethics,* edited by J. Burley and J. Harris, Maiden, Mass. Blackwell, pp. 245-252. Shalev C. (2002) 'Human Cloning and Human Rights: A Commentary', *Health and Human Rights,* 2002, 6 pp. 137-151; Schachter O. (1983) 'Human Dignity as a Normative Concept' *American Journal of International Law,* 77, pp. 848-854; Wright T.G. (2000) 'Second Thoughts: How Human Cloning Can Promote Human Dignity', *Valparaiso University Law Review*, 35, pp. 1-35.

(2) Gogarty B. (2003) 'What exactly is an exact copy? And why it matters when trying to ban reproductive cloning in Australia', *Journal of Medical Ethics*, 29, pp. 84-89.

(3) Gogarty B. (2003) 'What exactly is an exact copy? And why it matters when trying to ban reproductive cloning in Australia', *Journal of Medical Ethics*, 29, p. 84.

(4) Gogarty B. (2003) 'What exactly is an exact copy? And why it matters when trying to ban reproductive cloning in Australia', *Journal of Medical Ethics*, 29, p. 85.

(5)Gogarty B. (2003) 'What exactly is an exact copy? And why it matters when trying to ban reproductive cloning in Australia', *Journal of Medical Ethics*, 29, p. 87.

(6) I have argued elsewhere that even if people do have identical fingerprints, it is not known nor is it knowable either *a priori* or *a posteriori* that they do. It is unwarranted to say that each person must have a unique set of finger-prints (or, by the same reasoning, a unique set of genes or any other physical feature or arrangement of features). See McLachlan H.V., (1995), 'No Two Sets Exactly the Same? Applying Philosophy to the Theory of Fingerprints', *The Philosopher*, 83, pp. 12-18.

(7) See McLachlan, H.V., (2004) 'Human Embryos, Clones and Public Policy: A Critique of the Church of Scotland's Views', *Scottish Affairs*, 46, Winter.

(8) See Ridley, M., (2003) *Nature Via Nurture: Genes, Experience and What Makes Us Human*, London: Fourth Estate.

(9) Lederberg, J.., (2003) 'Learning from our complex relationship with bugs', *The Herald*, April 26, p. 15.

(10) Harris, J., (1997), '"Goodbye Dolly?" The Ethics of Human

Cloning', *Journal of Medical Ethics*, 23 p. 353.

(11) Mill, J.S., (1966), 'On Liberty', in Warnock, M., editor, *Utilitarianism*, London, Collins.

(12) See McLachlan, H.V. and Swales, J.K., (2001), 'Surrogate Motherhood, Rights and Duties: A Reply to Campbell', *Health Care Analysis*, 9, pp. 101-107.

(13) See, for instance, Advisers to the President of the European Commission on the Ethical Implications of Biotechnology, (1997), 'Ethical Aspects of Cloning Techniques', *Journal of Medical Ethics*, 23, pp. 349-352.

(14) That human cloning is against the will and purpose of God is also claimed by some as a reason for making human reproductive cloning illegal. I have considered and rejected this argument in 'Human Embryos, Clones and Public Policy: A Critique of the Church of Scotland's Views', *Scottish Affairs*, 46, Winter, 2004.

Chapter Eight

Bring on the Clones?

*Ignore The Boys from Brazil – say Yes to human cloning**

Human cloning is a notion that seems to horrify many people. For instance, a celebrated film – The Boys From Brazil – is based on the premise that the cloning of Hitler would be, for all decent people, an alarming prospect. It should not be. What should disturb and repel us is the popular prejudice against human clones and human cloning.

At present in the UK, human reproductive cloning is illegal. In terms of the Human Reproductive Cloning Act (2001): 'A person who places in a woman a human embryo which has been created otherwise than by fertilisation is guilty of an offence'. I think that this is thoroughly misguided and that the legislation should be repealed.

The very idea of human cloning and human clones is shocking to some people and seems to disturb their normal rational thought processes. Everything that can be done should be done, some people seem to think, to try to prevent the existence of human clones. They tend to argue that human cloning should be illegal because it is unethical and that it is unethical because it is the production of copies of individual persons, who should remain unique. Their argument is weak.

Not all unethical actions should be illegal. Even more so, not all actions that are thought to be unethical should, for that reason, be made illegal. Some people think that masturbation is unethical and one suspects that, but for the practicalities of the law enforcement concerned, they might want to make it a crime. In some instances at least, adultery is unethical even if it would be unwise to make it again, as it once was in Scotland, a crime. Human cloning as a technique and a form of asexual reproduction is no more inherently unethical than is normal sexual reproduction although particular instances of both can certainly be unethical. However, it does not follow that these particular unethical instances should be crimes. Even if, as a technique, human cloning were inherently unethical, it would not follow that it should thereby be made a crime.

In any case, we should distinguish between the clones and the cloning. Rape is and should be illegal. We do not, however, say that babies conceived by rape should not be born. Morally, such babies are no different from other babies. Although abortion is legally allowable in the event of conception that results from rape, we do not say that it should be legally compulsory. The moral status of persons as persons is independent of the biological and genealogical pedigree of their bodies. The law at present in relation to cloning stands in obscene defiance of this simple but profound truth.

Many of those who are against human cloning also argue against abortion and stem-cell research on the grounds of the interests and rights of embryos. Paradoxically, if they want to be consistent, they should also argue against the present law against cloning. Not all means to good ends are justified. Even if the prevention of human cloning were a good end, the present law would be unjustifiable as a means of producing it.

In any case, cloning does not involve the copying of individual persons. The central objection to human cloning is misplaced. Persons cannot be copied. Persons can have bodies but bodies are not persons. Cloning relates to the reproduction of bodies by means of replicating their genes.

Identical twins have identical sets of genes. They are not in any other sense identical. They are certainly not physically identical. For instance, they do not have identical fingerprints. Often, when we get to know them, we realise that even facially, they are readily distinguishable. Identical twins do not have identical personalities. Sometimes, they do not even have noticeably similar personalities. Genes are important but they are nothing like as causally important as they are commonly thought to be. We are not our genes. There is more to us than our physical bodies and more to our bodies than our genes. Identical twins are not identical persons.

People who are twins should be treated with the same moral respect as other people. They are the same as other people. Insofar as people are unique, each individual twin is unique. For instance, we are uniquely responsible for our own actions. We deserve praise when we do good things and the opposite when we do bad things. This is so for twins no more or less than for anyone else. It would be absurd to blame a person for something that his twin did.

What is true for twins is true for clones. People whose bodies were cloned from the bodies of other people are no less people than are other people. Insofar as people in general are unique, they are similarly unique. They are, for instance, responsible for their own actions no more or less than is any one else.

Suppose that it were to be discovered that Hitler had an identical twin called Helmut. If Helmut were still alive, it would be absurd to blame and punish him for the actions of his twin. He was not the author of these actions. Helmut might be a smashing bloke. There is no reason to assume that he would have the same personality as his twin. Even if he did have the same tastes and dispositions as Hitler, he might have made better choices with his life. Twins, no more or less than anyone else have freedom of the will.

Suppose that, from some fragment of Hitler's body, it was possible to form an embryonic human body with a set of genes identical to Hitler's body's genes. I don't for a moment imagine that this is a practical possibility but, for the sake of the argument, let us suppose that it were. If that embryo were to be allowed to develop in a woman's womb, it would become a loveable baby and, in time, the mature body of an adult human being. The person whose body it became would be due as much moral respect as persons are normally due. The person would be, in the same sense as we all are, unique. He would be responsible for his own actions. He, just like Helmut, would not be responsible for Hitler's actions. He, just like Helmut, might or might not be in character or temperament, like Hitler. If, say, he happens to be anti-Semitic, he might choose not to act upon such inclinations: he might repudiate them.

The present law against human reproductive cloning is unethical and irrational. It should be repealed. Sooner or later, there will be human clones. We should be ready to welcome them and love them, just as we would welcome and love other babies.

'Poor reasons for making human cloning illegal'**

Professor Haldane argues against my claim that human reproductive cloning should be legal. (*The Scotsman*, Science, 12th Nov) If his arguments were sound, then normal sexual intercourse between husbands and wives should often be a criminal offence. Fortunately, his arguments are unconvincing.

He writes that: 'Reproductive cloning is uncertain and unsafe'. It will not always succeed in producing living and undamaged embryos. This is true but irrelevant. It is one thing to risk causing damage to bodies that would otherwise be whole and healthy. It is something else to risk causing damage to embryos that, but for the risky action, would not exist.

When people have normal sexual intercourse in order to have babies, what they do is uncertain and unsafe. They are likely to fail. If they succeed in producing an embryo, it might well die. They run the risk of producing babies that are unhealthy and deformed.

The risk is higher in some instances than in others. Sometimes, the risk can be known in advance to be very high. However, it does not follow that it should be a crime to try to have babies. It will, perhaps, sometimes be unwise and sometimes unethical to do so but it should not be a crime.

The attitudes and motives of those people who want to have clones are suspect, according to Haldane. This, perhaps, is true in some cases but it is beside the point. The same might be said of people in general who want to have children. However, their motives for having children and their attitudes are their own business. The law should not intrude. What matters is how they treat children once they are born.

Another reason that Haldane gives for making cloning a criminal offence is the claim that the lives of clones will be hard to bear because some people will not give clones the respect that, as human beings, they deserve. The claim might be true. However, if this is a problem, it is a problem about such people not about clones or cloning. At some times and places it was illegal for black and white people to have sexual intercourse on the grounds that the resulting babies would be abnormal and not be given the same respect that normal human beings are given. This was a bad reason for making such procreative activities a criminal offence. Similarly, what Haldane suggests is a poor, unworthy reason for making human reproductive cloning illegal.

He suggests that, in the interests of possible clones, we should prevent their existence by making cloning illegal. This is a speculative and unconvincing argument. To say that it would be so unpleasant to be a clone that it would be better not to exist at all is implausible. Is it better not to be born at all than to be born deformed or disabled? Is it better not to be born at all than to have parents that have unreasonable and oppressive expectations about one's likely future achievements? Surely not.

*By Hugh V McLachlan from *The Scotsman*, 5th November 2005.

**By Hugh V McLachlan from *The Scotsman*, 26th November 2005.

Surrogate Motherhood

Chapter Nine

Commercial Surrogate Motherhood*

Surrogate motherhood and, in particular, commercial surrogate motherhood (C.S.M) has received much criticism and little support. This seems to us to be unfortunate. The case against surrogate motherhood, including commercial surrogate motherhood, is weaker than in commonly supposed.

Among the proposals of the *Report of the Committee of Inquiry into Human Fertilisation and Embryology* which were put into effect by the relevant legislation in 1990 was that commercial surrogate motherhood agreements and agencies should be illegal. This seems to have been popular legislation. Indeed, when, recently, a surrogate mother, who had been commissioned by a Dutch couple to carry a baby for them and who had received expenses for her services, changed her mind and decided to keep the baby (after lying about having had an abortion), the reaction of the press to this was curious. There was not only the expression of the view that the British legislation heads in the right direction but of the view that perhaps the legislation might be reconsidered in order – how? – to make it even tougher against surrogate motherhood and, in particular, commercial surrogate motherhood.

Perhaps there has been relatively little defence of C.S.M. because the issue is not one that is likely to affect many people directly. Nevertheless, for the people involved, the matter can be of considerable importance, particularly for the prospective parents, at least some of whom, in the absence of C.S.M., will not become parents and for the prospective children of whom, in the absence of C.S.M., most, or even all will not be born.

Some people might wonder why some other people should go to all the bother and expense of procuring a child *via* surrogate motherhood, especially when there already exist in the world children who are in need of parents. Some people might even consider that the commissioning parents in surrogate motherhood arrangements are being selfish or, at least, self-indulgent.

There are two responses we would make. First of all, if people want to enter into such arrangements, it is their own business: the law has no legitimate interests in the motives of the people involved. Secondly, it is no more selfish to want to become a parent with the aid of a surrogate mother than it is to want to become one in the normal way. If there are objections to introducing more children into an arguably over-populated world, then, again, these would apply generally to the production of children. They would have no particular or exclusive applicability to the case of children borne by commercial and (non-commercial) surrogate mothers.

It has been argued on two general grounds that C.S.M. should be illegal: because it is immoral and because it can cause problems and complications. Neither sort of argument is convincing.

Whether something is immoral and whether or not it is a good idea to make it illegal are separate questions. For instance, in the past in Scotland, adultery was a criminal offence. Indeed, it was (for flagrant and persistent occurrences) a capital offence. One might well agree that it is a good idea that adultery is no longer a crime without thereby being committed to the view that adultery is never immoral. Prohibition in America was a very, very bad idea. It was unwise to make the purchase and consumption of alcohol illegal no matter whether or not all or some of that purchase and consumption was immoral.

In any case, it is very far from clear that C.S.M. is immoral. Why should it be considered immoral? The main problem with the claim that C.S.M. is inherently immoral is that its proponents have not demonstrated that it is necessarily harmful, while it seems clear that all the parties involved, especially the resulting children who would not otherwise be born, could benefit from it.

Lady Warnock, who chaired the Committee of Inquiry into Human Fertilisation and Embryology, says that: 'Even if a calculation of benefits and harms were to show conclusively that the balance was in favour of permitting surrogacy, there would still remain many who would be left with the feeling that it was wrong all the same'. The implication seems to be that Warnock is such a person.

The crux of Warnock's case is that she and, she implies, most other people feel revulsion at the thought of C.S.M. We do not share Warnock's revulsion nor are we convinced that C.S.M. is immoral. Whose views are more representative, Warnock's or ours? We do not know. In any case, mere distaste or revulsion does not seem in itself a good reason for restricting the freedom of action of other people especially where these other people do not share that distaste or revulsion.

An argument sometimes used here is that C.S.M. is morally wrong because it is morally wrong to buy and sell babies since this involves treating human beings as mere commodities, which is wrong. Sometimes too it is suggested that C.S.M. involves treating the carrying mother as a commodity.

These arguments seem to us to be weak ones. It would certainly be wrong to buy and sell babies if the consequence was that bought and sold babies were treated like the inanimate objects which are normally bought and sold. It is wrong to treat people, in all respects, as if they were inanimate objects whether or not they were, as babies, bought and sold.

What does it mean to say that C.S.M. involves buying a baby? If you buy, say, a house or a motor car, then you have legal rights and duties concerning that motor car which others do not have. If you 'buy' a baby, what rights and duties do you have which differ from those which parents have towards their children who were born in the normal way? Children acquired as a result of C.S.M. do not become inanimate objects. C.S.M. is neither a form of nor a basis for slavery.

In any case, it seems whimsical to say that commercial surrogate motherhood involves the buying and selling of *babies*. What is bought and sold are *the services of the carrying mother*. If you pay a taxi-driver to convey your body and your baby's body from one place to another or, as you might do in some cultures and circumstances, if you pay a porter to carry you and/or your baby from one place to another, you are not thereby involved in some sort of immoral action. You are not treating the taxi-driver or the porter or your own body or your baby's body as a mere commodity.

Why is the surrogate mother not worthy of her hire? There is an obvious opportunity cost involved in the rendering of her services. Why does payment in recompense for this cost have anything to do with treating the woman or the baby as a mere commodity? We do not think that it does any more than does, say, paying journalists for what they, with their minds and bodies, produce implies treating them as commodities.

Just as it can be a good idea not to make some immoral actions crimes, sometimes it is a good idea to make some particular actions illegal even though they are not inherently immoral. For instance, it is not inherently immoral to drive motor cars on the left nor on the right hand side of the road but it can be advisable to create laws about what side of the road should be favoured for normal driving.

Even if C.S.M. is not immoral, perhaps it should be illegal? Perhaps, as its opponents suggest, it should be illegal because of the problems it can and could create?

Various things in life cause problems and complications. This is not in itself much of an argument for making them crimes. For instance, marriage causes complications and problems as does having, even in the normal way, children. How many people regret having married and/or regret having had children (or regret *not* having had children)? Plenty of them. Should marriage on that account be made illegal? Should the having of children (or the failure to have children) become criminal offences? Hardly! Surrogate motherhood arrangements (whether commercial or not) can undoubtedly cause problems. For instance, after parting with and from a carried child, a carrying mother might be regretful. She might experience deep trauma. However, such evidence as there is suggests that such regret and trauma are not inevitable. Furthermore, if it is adult, informed women who voluntarily become surrogate mothers, the fact that some of them might later regret it hardly seems much of a justification for outlawing the practice. Some women regret having had abortions. Some women regret not having had abortions. Some women regret having married. Some women regret not having married. Such is life.

A potentially more serious problem is the welfare of the children involved. If such children were shown to have unhappy lives or to feel that they bore some sort of a social stigma, then we would certainly be prepared to change our views on C.S.M. However, there seems to us to be no *prima facia* case for thinking that this would be their likely lot in life.

There are potential legal complications concerning the parentage of the children involved. Suppose, say, that the commissioning parents are also the genetic parents of a child who is carried by another woman. This might happen in a situation where a woman is not infertile but is prevented from carrying a child by, for instance, a deformity of the womb. Who is or should be the legal mother of the child? What if the carrying mother changes her mind and does not want to part with the child, does not want to give the child to the commissioning couple of whom at least one might be the genetic parent of the child? What should happen? We do not know how these questions should be answered. Nonetheless, we imagine that the law could evolve, as it has done in the past, to deal reasonably with novel situations and issues.

Some people express the fear that, sometimes, none of the parties involved might want to accept a child born of a surrogate mother. In particular, they ask: 'What if such a child is born handicapped or deformed?' Well, what do most parents do if, in the normal way, they produce a handicapped or deformed child? Do they not love and care for it? Why should commissioning parents be expected to behave differently? Furthermore, if through death or whatever, the children involved are not cared for by the commissioning parents or the carrying mothers, there are social services and potential foster and adoptive parents to look after them and the number of such children is likely to be small. Perhaps, too, it might be possible to plan for the special needs of such disabled children even more readily than for those of disabled children born in the normal way through, say, putting a levy on the fees for all C.S.M. and placing the money thereby raised into a special insurance fund. Legalisation might allow for the possibility of regulation and control of C.S.M. and of the problems it can produce.

With surrogate motherhood and perhaps particularly with commercial surrogate motherhood, there is the danger that one or other of the parties involved will be exploited. There is the danger, for instance, that commissioning parents will pay money for the services of a surrogate mother and not receive the services they have paid for. The carrying mother might keep or abort the baby. Similarly, the surrogate mother might deliver the baby, in more senses than one, and fail to receive sufficient money or, possibly, any money at all for her services. There are potential problems with all commercial contracts. Obviously, to make all commercial contracts illegal would not be a satisfactory solution to that general problem.

There are too, perhaps, various other potential problems with commercial surrogate motherhood and surrogate motherhood as such of which we are unaware (just as there might well be various other benefits of which we and the opponents of surrogate motherhood fail to allow for). However, we do not think that these problems are insurmountable or that they are best dealt with by making and keeping commercial surrogate motherhood arrangements and agencies illegal. Indeed, the illegality of surrogate motherhood makes some of these problems more severe. The parties directly affected are more likely to be exploited when commercial surrogate motherhood is illegal than they would be were it to be legalised. The commissioning parents in particular are likely to be exploited when C.S.M. is illegal. The illegalisation is almost bound to increase the cost of C.S.M. They run the risk of paying for the services of carrying mothers yet failing to be provided with the anticipated babies. Where C.S.M. arrangements are illegal, commissioning parents cannot be legally compensated for such breaches of contract. Furthermore, it is undesirable that children are born under a cloud of illegality as some will be with the illegalisation of C.S.M..

The problems of C.S.M. do not automatically disappear by making C.S.M. illegal. Indeed, the problems of illegal C.S.M. might well be greater than the problems of C.S.M. (just as in America, the 'solution' of Prohibition caused more problems than did the drunkenness, whose problems it was supposed to solve). However, if commercial surrogate motherhood agencies and agreements are completely unacceptable – although we do not see why they should be – there are alternatives to simply outlawing organised surrogate motherhood. Perhaps current fostering and adoption agencies suggest possible exemplars.

*By Hugh V. McLachlan and J. Kim Swales, from *Contemporary Review*, 1998, March, Vol. 272, No. 1586, pp. 113-117.

Chapter Ten

Babies, Child Bearers and Commodification: Anderson, Brazier *et. al.* and the Political Economy of Commercial Surrogate Motherhood.*

Abstract.

It is argued by Anderson and also in the Brazier Report that Commercial Surrogate Motherhood (C.S.M.) contracts and agencies should be illegal on the grounds that C.S.M. involves the commodification of both mothers and babies. This paper takes issue with this view and argues that C.S.M. is not inconsistent with the proper respect for, and treatment of, children and women. A case for the legalisation of C.S.M. is made.

Key words: commodification, Commercial Surrogate Motherhood, surrogacy, Brazier Report, medical ethics

Introduction

Anderson (1993) argues – forcefully, and in terms of her impressive pluralistic theory of value – that not everything that could be should be available for sale on the market. In this general claim, we are in agreement with her. However, when she says that, in particular, commercial surrogate motherhood (C.S.M) should be illegal, she is less convincing.

It is not against commercial surrogate mothers themselves that Anderson directs her attack but against commercial surrogate motherhood agencies and, to an extent, against commissioning parents. Anderson writes: 'Because the surrogate mother is one of the victims of contract pregnancy, she should not be prosecuted for entering into the contract. My arguments are directed only against surrogacy as a commercial enterprise, not as a pure gift relationship' (Anderson, 1993, footnote 9: 229).

At the kernel of Anderson's case lies the notion of 'commodification'. Anderson says:

'... contract pregnancy commodities both women's labor and children in ways that undermine the autonomy and dignity of women and the love parents owe to their children. Because the state has a legitimate interest in protecting the autonomy and dignity of women and the integrity of parental love for children, it is justified in prohibiting contract pregnancy.' (Anderson, 1993: 168)

Anderson presents other suggested related objections to C.S.M.

or, as it is also called, 'contract pregnancy' – that it reinforces gender inequality and is exploitative of commercial surrogate mothers – but we shall focus here specifically on her argument about commodification.

Anderson says: 'At the very least, pregnancy contracts should not be enforceable. Mothers should not be forced to relinquish children with whom they have formed emotional bonds' (Anderson, 1993: 186). She says too: 'The ethical objections raised against contract pregnancy even support the stronger conclusion that commercial surrogate contracts should be illegal and that surrogate agencies which arrange such contracts should be subject to criminal penalties' (Anderson, 1993: 186).

Similar policy conclusions are made for similar reasons in the recent Brazier Report on Surrogacy.[1] The Brazier Report recommended that surrogate mothers should be paid, by commissioning parents, only in regard to actual expenses caused by the pregnancy. It recommended the continuation of Section 1A of the 1985 Surrogacy Act whereby the non-enforceability of surrogate motherhood contracts (and not merely commercial ones) was specified.

In the report, it is written:

'We recommend the enactment of a new Surrogacy Act to ban payments other than expenses, to require the registration of surrogacy agencies and to give statutory force to a Code of Practice. Contraventions of the ban on payments to the surrogate [mother] other than expenses would result in ineligibility for a parental order. It would become a criminal offence to operate an unregistered surrogacy agency.' (Brazier *et al.*, 1998: ii)

Only 'non-profit making' surrogate motherhood agencies would be allowed to be registered. The advertising of both commercial and non-commercial surrogate motherhood provisions and arrangements would be illegal.

The reasons offered for these recommendations overlap with some of those given by Anderson for hers. The report says:

'We find that payments to surrogate mothers, other than in recompense for genuine expenses, give rise to the following concerns.

(1) Payments create a danger that women will give less than free and fully informed consent to act as a surrogate.

(2) Payments risk the commodification of the child to be born.

(30 Payments contravene the social norms of our society that, just as bodily parts cannot be sold, nor can such intimate services.'

(Brazier *et al.*, 1998: i)

We shall consider here, since they pertain to commodification, the suggested arguments (2) and (3) against C.S.M.

Anderson and Brazier argue that there are ethical objections concerning 'commodification' to C.S.M. and that it should be illegal. We shall suggest that it is not thus ethically objectionable and that, even if it were, it should not on that account be made or kept illegal: the public policy proposals of Anderson and of Brazier are not well served by the arguments about 'commodification' which they tender in their support. We do not accept that C.S.M. involves the 'commodification' (in a sense of wrongly treating them as objects) of either babies or women. Consider, first of all, the alleged commodification of babies.

C.S.M. and the Alleged Commodification of Babies

Anderson thinks that C.S.M. degrades children and disrespects their inherent moral worth as human beings. It, she says, '... constitutes a degrading traffic in children ...' (Anderson, 1993: 186). She writes that: 'In selling children, the parties to contract pregnancy express attitudes towards children that contradict the norms of parental love. They accept the legitimacy of paying mothers to undermine their love for their children' (Anderson, 1993: 172). She argues that, if C.S.M. became common, it could:

'... psychologically threaten all children ... For it would change the way people (parents and brokers) value children generally – from being worthy of love by their parents and respect by others, to being sometimes the alienated objects of commercial profit making.' (Anderson, 1993: 172)

We would argue that C.S.M. is not the buying and selling of babies and, furthermore, whether or not it is, it does not have the implications and consequences which Anderson claims that it has. Kornegay (1990) is nearer the mark, we think, in suggesting that commissioning parents pay the surrogate mother for the services of carrying and delivering the baby rather than for the baby itself. What the commissioning parents pay for as well, and this seems often to be overlooked, is the entrepreneurial services of the C.S.M. agency in bringing together the surrogate mother and commissioning parents and otherwise helping to facilitate the arrangement.

Parents might own their sperm and their eggs. They might even own their embryos but they do not own the children whose bodies such embryos might become; nor do they own the bodies of such children. (Whether people even own their own bodies is a complex and unclear issue (see McLachlan, 1997 a).) Parental rights, as Arneson and van Nierkerk and van Zyl (1995) convincingly argue are not property rights. Babies are not property and should not (and cannot) be treated in all respects like property. C.S.M. does not imply that they are property or that they will necessarily be treated as if they were. Parents are not legally entitled to treat and dispose of their children in the ways – and they are not the same in all cases – in which they are entitled to treat and dispose of those things which they legally own. This leads Arneson and van Nierkerk and van Zyl to consider that parents do not own their children, however they acquire them.

We think that van Nierkerk and van Zyl are correct when they say: 'The surrogacy agreement cannot be compared to the act of going shopping for a new car. When paying someone to be a surrogate mother, one does not thereby buy the right to treat the child as an object' (van Niekerk and van Zyl, 1995a: 167). Furthermore, C.S.M. does not imply that parties to the agreement will treat it as an object for their own us '... any more than if parents had a child in the conventional way' (van Niekerk and van Zyl, 1995a: 168).

Suppose that you own, say, property in a house. Now, you can sell this to someone else. There would be a flow of money from the other person to you and there would be a corresponding transfer of the bundle of legal rights and duties which constitute ownership of the particular house from you to the other person.[2] This is different from what happens with C.S.M. Suppose that the surrogate mother gives a baby to the commissioning parents, who give the surrogate mother money. No bundle of legal rights and duties to or concerning the baby has flowed from the surrogate mother to the commissioning parents precisely because the baby is not a commodity and C.S.M. cannot turn it into one.

Children are not property and hence the question of buying and selling them does not arise. van Niekerk and van Zyl go on to say: 'But we would like to suggest that what is being sold by the surrogate in cases of commercial surrogacy is not the child, but the right to be regarded as the child's parent' (van Niekerk and van Zyl, 1995a: 168-169). It is not clear that this latter suggestion is quite right. It is not clear that parental rights any more than, for instance, a driving licence or the legal obligation to serve, on conviction, a prison sentence could or should be bought and sold. Furthermore, it would seem to conflict with their other claim that: 'The surrogate merely agrees to a contract in which she relinquishes her right to claim legal parenthood of the ensuing child' (van Niekerk and van Zyl, 1995a: 169).

In any event, van Niekerk and van Zyl would seem to us to be correct in maintaining that Anderson's argument does not hold and that objection cannot be made, in the way that she makes it, to C.S.M. on the grounds that it treats babies inappropriately as 'commodities', as objects of use rather than as moral ends in themselves as a Kantian might say. As van Niekerk and van Zyl say: 'Market norms do not in any way have to exclude the norms of parental love. Treating something as a commodity need not mean treating it *merely* or *only* as a commodity' (van Niekerk and van Zyl, 1995a: 168).

Consider, for example, cats. Even if they are not due the same respect as human beings are, it would be wrong, in some contexts, to treat them in ways in which it might be proper to treat some particular commodities. For instance, in some contexts, it would be proper to set fire to a piece of coal but improper to set fire to a cat. However, it is not wrong to purchase both pieces of coal and cats. It is not wrong to treat cats and coal in the same way in some respects: it depends on the respects. Do people who pay money to purchase, as kittens, expensive pedigree cats treat them worse than those people treat their cats who acquire them, say, as strays or as gifts? Of course not. They often treat them better.

Similarly, it is not necessarily wrong to treat human beings in some respects in the same way that one treats a commodity. It depends on the treatment; it depends on the respect in which it is the same. Not *all* treatment which might be appropriate for a commodity would be appropriate for a human being; but that is another matter.

In response to Arneson's observation that parents of children acquired through C.S.M, just like other parents, do not acquire unlimited rights to do whatever they might want to do to the children concerned, Anderson says that:

'This shows that children transferred by pregnancy contracts are not completely commodified, as slaves are. But they are still partially commodified in that the contract permits parents to transfer rights to custody in their children for profit.' (Anderson, 1993: 171-172)

In our view, Anderson misses the point here. Babies acquired as the result of C.S.M. are not 'partial commodities'. They are certainly not partial slaves. They are no more slaves than are babies of a normal background. Even if it were true, we do not say it is but even if it were true, that they were treated in one respect in the same way as commodities are, that would not make them 'partial commodities'. Nor would the treatment necessarily be wrong. Some commodities are cherished, cleaned and insured. It is not wrong to cherish, clean and insure babies.

Consider Anderson's slave analogy further. Imagine that the only way in which it was possible to free a particular slave was to buy him and give him his freedom. Would the purchase of such a slave and the treatment of him in one respect as a commodity be wrong? We do not think so. With some particular children, the only possibility of their birth and existence lies in their being involved in a C.S.M. arrangement. If they were treated as a commodity in this one and only respect that payment was made for them it is far from clear that such treatment would be wrong.

As already stated, it is also the view of Brazier *et al.* that: 'Payments risk the commodification of the child to be born' (1998: i). Furthermore, we noted that this argument is not convincing. It does not follow that a child need nor will be treated merely as a commodity nor in ways inappropriate for a child to be treated if payment is made to the women who carried him before his birth. Note too that payment by the commissioning parents *to a commercial surrogate motherhood agency* for their entrepreneurial services clearly does not constitute the improper treatment as a commodity of the baby concerned. After all, some people pay, and quite properly pay, dating agencies and matrimonial agencies for their services in bringing together potential partners. When marriages result from introductions thus effected and when children are produced in such marriages people do not claim – do they? – that the relevant spouses and children were purchased or are necessarily in any other inappropriate respects treated as commodities.

The writers of the report, when indicating their concern about 'commodification' and child-bearing, consider the argument that payment is made for the services of carrying the baby rather than for the baby itself and say:

'We find it difficult to see how this distinction can be maintained, especially because any fully commercialised contract of this kind should be subject to the normal laws of contract. It is unimaginable that a commissioning couple should enter into a contract that required simply that the surrogate [mother] became pregnant and gave birth. The contract would have to contain a requirement that in return for the fee, the child would be handed over to those contracting the pregnancy, with penalties for failure to fulfil this aspect of the agreement.' (1998: 38)

Now, there is something in what Brazier *et al.* say here insofar as it is true to say that when commissioning parents pay a surrogate mother, they *expect* to receive something other than the knowledge that a baby has been carried: they might even *imagine* that they have purchased a particular baby. However, what they do expect and imagine is one thing and what they should expect and imagine might be something else. What they have paid for is not necessarily the same as what they think they have paid for. What they want the surrogate mother and the surrogate motherhood agency to give them and what they could and will be given can diverge. What they think they have bought will not necessarily correspond to what the surrogate mother and the surrogate motherhood agency think that they have sold.

C.S.M. and the Alleged Commodification of Women and/ or of their Bodies

Consider now women and/or their child-bearing labour in relation to commodification. According to Anderson:

'Contract pregnancy transforms what is specifically women's labor – the work of bringing forth children into the world – into a commodity.... The application of commercial norms to women's reproductive labor reduces surrogate mothers from persons worthy of respect and consideration to dominated objects of mere use.' (Anderson, 1993: 175)

This is not at all convincing. The bringing forth of children into the world is not merely a commodity: nothing can transform it into a mere commodity. To treat it in some respect like a mere commodity, for example, by giving payment for it, need not at all be to fail to allow for the various respects in which it is unlike most commodities and unlike all mere commodities.

Women who are surrogate mothers are, as human beings, due as much respect as anyone else. Presumably, Anderson does not want to deny this. Is she saying, rather, that, as a matter of fact, (some) people do not treat women who are surrogate mothers with the dignity and respect which they are due? This might be true but if it is, it indicates a problem not about surrogate motherhood but one about these particular people. What can be done to help them? Anderson's comments seem particularly unhelpful in this regard. Anderson writes:

'Few things reach deeper into the self than a parent's evolving relationship with her own child. Laying claim to the course of this relationship in virtue of a cash payment constitutes a severe violation of the mother's personhood and a denial of her autonomy.'

(Anderson, 1993: 178)

It is not at all clear that this argument has much force. If people are 'laying claim' to the course of this relationship, they are not doing so 'by virtue of a cash payment' but by virtue of the fact that the surrogate mother (through an exercise of her moral autonomy) consented to enter into a relationship which involved giving these people a legitimate interest and possibly a say in the course of her pregnancy. If the state disallows such relationships then it can hardly do so on the grounds of the protection of the autonomy of the prospective surrogate mother. Sometimes, as for example in the case of minors, the state tries to protect people from the undesirable consequences to them of their own actions but this is justified – when it is justified – precisely because minors are not considered to be fully morally autonomous beings.

The surrogate mother who enters into a C.S.M. contract (or any other contract) will, in some respects, not be as autonomous as she would be if she had not done so. That is what a contract is. Because she is autonomous, she can enter into agreements and relationships but it is a consequence of such entry that she will not have in all respects the autonomy which she would have had had she chosen not to do so. If she is pregnant and chooses to get married, she does not retain the autonomy to have the perspective on her life and pregnancy that she might have had had she not got married. Surrogate motherhood is similar. Part of our freedom is the authority, sometimes in unpredicted and even unpredictable ways, voluntarily to limit, our autonomy.[3] If a woman chooses to 'violate her personhood and limit her autonomy' by becoming a commercial surrogate mother, then it would be a violation of her personhood and a denial of her autonomy – it seems to us – to disallow her to become one.

Although van Niekerk and van Zyl do not think that C.S.M is 'intrinsically immoral' with regard to the baby, they think that, for the reason of inappropriate commodification, it is immoral 'from the perspective of the surrogate mother herself. Their case, however, is not a strong one. They state:

'The problem with surrogacy arrangements is therefore that it causes a woman to be pregnant while expecting her not to acknowledge the fact that she is expecting her child. It tries to divorce pregnancy from the conscious knowledge that you are going to give birth to *your* child. In this way the surrogate becomes a mere 'environment' or 'human incubator' for someone else's child.' (van Niekerk and van Zyl, 1995b: 347)

Consider, in particular, gestational surrogate motherhood, i.e. where the surrogate mother carries the fertilised egg of the commissioning woman. Here, the surrogate mother is and she clearly is, a human incubator for someone else's child but she is not 'merely' a human incubator nor a 'mere environment'. She is also an autonomous moral agent who is worthy of moral respect. Similarly, a woman who, after the normal fashion, becomes and remains pregnant is an environment for and a human incubator for a child who is her child and the child of her partner but there is no reason, just as there is no reason in the case of a commercial surrogate mother, to think of her as being a *mere* environment nor a *mere* human incubator.

According to van Niekerk and van Zyl:

'... Anderson's point is not that surrogacy is immoral because it is a form of alienated labour, but *because pregnancy should not become an act of alienated labour*. Being denied the legitimacy of one's perspective on one's labour, being alienated from your feelings and having to act against one's emotions is not wrong *per se*, but only wrong if the labour in question is women's reproductive labour (or another special form of labour). It is in this sense that surrogacy is similar to prostitution: not that both are forms of alienated labour, but that in both cases a physical capacity (sexual intercourse and gestation) that should be afforded special respect is degraded to a form of alienated labour.' (1995b: 345)

Whether or not C.S.M. is immoral for the reason which they indicate, it is not at all clear why van Niekerk and van Zyl think that it is a good idea to make C.S.M. illegal.[4] For instance, do they consider that the illegalisation of prostitution has been a successful policy where such a policy has been pursued? If this is the case, why do they think like this?

In any case, they do not demonstrate that C.S.M. is immoral for the reasons they indicate. It is not true, for instance, that C.S.M. denies women their 'legitimate perspective' on their own pregnancies. If people voluntarily become surrogate mothers then they might thereby alter what is the 'legitimate perspective' on their pregnancy but what is wrong with that? It might well be unwise for particular women or even for women in general to become commercial surrogate mothers but that is not the same as saying that C.S.M. is immoral or the same as saying that it should be illegal. When people, for instance, get married, then, thereafter, they might be said often to be constrained to act contrary to their feelings and inclination and to be denied the freedom to interpret and lead their own lives as they might otherwise see fit. This hardly seems much of a case for saying that marriage should be considered as an immoral institution nor for saying that it should be made illegal albeit that the bonds of marriage are likely to be far stronger and tighter than any commercial surrogate motherhood contract would prove to be.

Brazier *et al.* state, *a propos* of C.S.M. that: 'Payments contravene the social norms of our society that, just as bodily parts cannot be sold, nor can such intimate services' (Brazier *et al.*, 1998: i). This is a curious thing to say in the context. The point is: what are the *arguments* for and against making C.S.M. illegal? To make a claim about what the 'norms of our society' happen to be does not in itself constitute the making of a relevant argument.

Furthermore, it is very far from clear that the view that bodily parts and services should not be legally allowed to be bought and sold is anything like universally accepted in the UK. Consider the evidence which Brazier *et al.* present themselves in this connection. In the questionnaire which was formulated and distributed in connection with their Report, Brazier *et al.* did not even bother to include a question on people's attitudes towards the buying and selling of bodily parts and services as such. This question was included: 'Should payments [to surrogate mothers] include remuneration by way of payments for carrying the child?' About 60% of respondents answered: 'Yes'. Most respondents further specified that such remuneration should *not* be limited only to actual expenses incurred. (Note that Brazier *et al.* take the astonishing step of also presenting – as if they were more authentic? – the results of the replies to their questionnaire when the responses of those people who are reckoned by Brazier *et al.* to be associated with C.O.T.S. (Childlessness Overcome Through Surrogacy) are eliminated.)

Brazier *et al.* ask the questions, which they want to be answered, respectively, 'No' and 'Yes': '...is payment to the surrogate [mother] for her services acceptable? Do payments contravene ethical values ...?' (p. 30). Now, of course, C.S.M. is acceptable to some people and unacceptable to others. It is in accord with the values of some people and not in accord with the values of others. All this is beside the point. They go on to say:

'We believe that the core value here, on which many social arrangements in the United Kingdom are based, including blood and live organ donation, is the "gift relationship". It appears that, as a society, we believe that the use of our procreative capacities to assist others should also be a gift, not a commercial transaction.... We believe that surrogacy should be informed by the same values.' (pp. 39, 45)

These are assertions of their own views rather than arguments for them, far less arguments against opposing ones. What, in effect, Brazier *et al.* are saying here is that they would prefer it if their own views were to be accepted rather than rejected.

It is not clear that 'we as a society' believe what Brazier *et al.* say we believe. Furthermore, even if 'we as a society' believe or value such and such, other societies and other people do not. Perhaps they are right and 'we as a society' are wrong: the point is to look at the arguments not the 'values'. The ethical issue is not about what any person or category of persons happens to value. One ought to value highly that which is morally good whether one does or not. Britain, like any society, is a 'multi-values' one. For those people who happen to share the 'values' of Brazier *et al.*, there is no problem: they need not be nor use the services of commercial surrogate mothers. The problem arises for the rest of us. The issue is this: what is the justification for making commercial surrogate motherhood illegal when not everyone agrees that it should be illegal and some people might want to be, or to use the services of, commercial surrogate mothers? Talk of 'norms', 'values' and 'beliefs' fails to connect with this issue.

Note, in passing, the following rhetorical ploy. Brazier *et al.* state: '... some of our recommendations, particularly with regard to payments, go against the deeply held and very genuine opinions of some ... organisations (notably COTS)' (pp. 58-59). Is the reader to believe that what Brazier *et al.* say is based on 'values' while what others say, when it is opposed to this, is mere 'opinion'? Perhaps, then, the 'values' of Brazier *et al.* here are wrong and the 'opinions' of C.O.T.S. are true.

Public Policy Recommendations

Our recommendations are that:

(i) Commercial surrogate motherhood agreements should not be illegal; they should be legally recognised and legally enforceable. Commissioning parents who pay surrogate mothers a fee, of whatever amount, should not be penalised by being deprived of a parental order for a child or in any other way.

(ii) Commercial surrogate motherhood agencies should be legal. It should not be illegal to be a commercial surrogate motherhood agent. It should not be illegal to advertise nor otherwise promote the activities of such agents and agencies. Such agencies should be allowed to make a profit (and, if it so turns out, a loss). Such agents should be allowed to make a living from their activity as agents.

We shall elaborate on the recommendations.

With regard to (i), C.S.M. is the purchase of the services of a carrying mother. It is, arguably, the purchase of more than that although it is a matter or reasonable debate what, precisely, the additional factor is or additional factors are. As we have previously been led by the observations of Brazier *et al.* to note, what commissioning parents think they have bought and what commercial surrogate mothers and/or agencies think they have sold can diverge. This, contrary to the suggestions of Brazier *et al.*, is actually a good reason for the legality and legal recognition of specified commercial surrogate motherhood contracts. We think that the commissioning parents should be thought -reasonably or morally, if you like – to be buying her services in carrying the child for the commissioning couple and also to be buying from the surrogate mother her refraining from pursuing her claim for the legal custody and parenthood of the child in addition to her physical surrendering of it and that commercial surrogate motherhood contracts should be legally formulated on that basis.

The commissioning parents expect to get custody of the child and to be the child's legal parents. Their expectations might of might not be well founded. They are not purchasing either from the surrogate mother or from the surrogate motherhood agency (or from anyone else or any thing else) the custody of the child or the child. Neither the child nor the custody of the child is the property of the surrogate mother or the surrogate motherhood agency. Hence neither can be bought or sold whatever the parties to any such imagined transaction might think.

The courts grant but do not sell the custody of children, nor do they sell parenthood. Consider an imaginary analogy. Suppose that, for some reason or other, only one driving licence was available to be given out and that there were two people who had a claim to be given a driving licence. If one of them could be prevailed upon not to pursue his claim then the effect might be that the other person was given a driving licence. Whatever the result might be, this would not be the same thing as the purchase by this latter person of a licence whether or not money was used to induce the first person to refrain from the pursuit of the claim. The person received a licence because of the soundness of his claim to be given one.

Similarly, if two people have a claim to be given custody of a particular child and/or to be considered as the legal mother of him and one of them withdraws her claim and the other woman has her claim upheld, this is not precisely the same as the purchase of the right to custody and/or parenthood of the child. It is not, for example, like an auction where a higher bidder could come along and secure the spoils.

It should be made clear to the commissioning parents that it might turn out that they are not given custody of the child and/or that they might not become the legal parents of the child. They run a risk. In the contractual agreement it should be specified what should happen concerning the fee in the event that the surrogate mother and the agency fulfil their sides of the bargain and yet the commissioning parents do not end up with the legal custody and/or parenthood of the child.

Those who say that marriage should be legally allowable and legally recognised do not necessarily say that divorce should be illegal or that reluctant husbands and wives should be physically forced to live together. Similarly, those who, like us, are in favour of legalised commercial surrogate motherhood arrangements do not necessarily imply that a surrogate mother who changes her mind mid-term and wants to keep the child should be forced to do, come what may, what she agreed to do and that, if necessary, the baby should be dragged from her breast by burly policemen. No: contracts can be broken although not always with impunity or without consequences.

Furthermore, marriage – although, it strictly speaking does not constitute a legal contract; rather, it relates to the status of two people and the nature of their relationship – suggests how such surrogate motherhood contracts might be formulated. People who are contemplating marriage to each other sometimes enter into (in some jurisdictions)legally enforceable pre-nuptial contractual agreements wherein it is specified what will be expected to happen in the event that one or other of the parties changes his or her mind after the marriage has begun and wants to discontinue it. A similar arrangement could be part of the commercial surrogate motherhood contract. Such contracts could (and should) specify what the agreed outcomes will be in the event that one or more of the parties has a subsequent change of heart.

Brazier *et al.* state:

'It is possible to imagine a new legislative framework, which permitted payment of a fee to the surrogate [mother], whilst maintaining her right to retain the child, but any such legislation would rationally have to contain provision for the contracting couple to obtain redress in the event that the child was not handed over. These legal considerations lead us to the conclusion that any financial arrangement that involves remuneration rather than simply expenses has to be regarded as a form of child purchase.' (p. 38)

This in not convincing. The redress concerned might simply be the return of any fee which had already been paid. It might be the return of the fee plus compensation. This would not be the purchase of a child. It could not even be reasonably misinterpreted, it seems to us, as the purchase of a child. Even if it were the purchase of a child, as long as the child were treated subsequently as a child should be treated, then the 'commodification' involved might be excusable or, even, laudable. Brazier *et al.* seem to be bemused by the idea of money changing hands and to be misled by this bemusement into drawing false conclusions about the nature and effects of financial transactions.

Consider again the slavery analogy. What was wrong with slavery, one might say, was not that money changed hands – it was not that people were bought and sold – but that people were, and were treated as, slaves. They lacked the legal rights of normal citizens and were denied – although they possessed them – the moral rights of human beings. Would slavery have been less reprehensible if 'commercial' slavery had been illegal and, rather than being bought and sold, slaves were always given and accepted as gifts? No, it would not.

The case of babies is similar. The crucial issue is how, once acquired, they are treated. Whether or not money changes hands in relation to this acquisition is not pivotal. Imagine some society where biological parents were not given the custody of their own children until they had paid a 'baby tax'. Babies and people in general might be treated just as well in that society as people are in contemporary Britain: they might be treated better. Overall, such a society might be a far better one than contemporary Britain (good though it is) is.

Regarding (ii), C.S.M. agencies serve the useful function of liaising with commissioning couples and surrogate mothers. Without this service, in most cases they would not even come into effective contact. It is quite appropriate that a fee is paid to agencies, whether by the commissioning couple or by the surrogate mother, for this service. The agencies too, in mediating between commissioning parents and surrogate mothers, might do other useful things for which payment is not inappropriate. For instance, they can act as advisers, referees, counsellors and listeners to complaints, queries and comments. Furthermore, they can hold, in such a form and place that reference can conveniently be made to them, definitive versions of the surrogacy contracts.

Note that, despite what Brazier *et al.* might suggest – and it is surprising and unfortunate that a Team to Review the arrangements regarding payment to surrogate mothers had no economists in it – whether or not an organisation is 'profit-making' is a different question than whether or not the organisation is 'commercial'. For instance, a building society might be transformed from a statutory non-profit making institution into a profit or loss making bank without becoming any more or less commercial in its operations.

Note too that Brazier *et al.* seem confused about what is signified by an organisation's being or not being 'profit-making'. For instance, universities charge fees and they pay their employees wages, in some cases generous wages, whether or not they are 'profit-making' and whether or not they are, as they can be, registered charities. The difference between these various statuses would seem to be matters of accountancy rather than of ethical principle. In any event, whether people make a living from, say, education or C.S.M. is a different matter from whether or not they make a profit from it.

With regard to (i) and (ii), there can be further specifications of the desirable legal context of C.S.M. once it is agreed that the related agencies should be legal. To say that it should be legal is not to say that it should be unregulated. On the contrary, it is illegal commercial surrogate motherhood agreements and agencies rather than legal ones which are likely to be anarchical. As the experience of Prohibition well proves, to make a commercial activity illegal is not the same as stopping it. As the experience well proves too, black markets are troublesome. If the 'commodification' of babies and surrogate mothers were undesirable then, how much more so, one might think, would be their illegal 'commodification'. Herein lies the practical political issue which needs to be faced. The relevant question is not whether the buying and selling of the services pertaining to surrogate motherhood is unethical but – given that these services will continue to be bought and sold (even if to a reduced extent) if trade in them is criminalised – whether it is better that they are bought and sold on the open or on the black market.

Conclusion

Anderson says: 'The case of contract pregnancy raises deep questions about the proper scope of the market in modern industrial societies' and she continues:

'... there are principled grounds for rejecting the substitution of market norms for parental norms to govern the ways women bring children into the world. When market norms are applied to the ways we allocate and understand parental rights and responsibilities over children, children are reduced from the subjects of respect and consideration to the objects of use. When market norms are applied to the ways we treat and understand women's reproductive labor, women are reduced from subjects of respect and consideration to objects of use.' (Anderson, 1993: 189)

She concludes that: 'If we are to retain the capacity to value children and women in ways consistent with their rightful claims to respect and consideration, we must resist the encroachment of the market into the sphere of reproductive labor' (Anderson, 1993: 189). We think, and we have shown why we think, that this conclusion is false. C.S.M. is not inconsistent with the proper respect for and treatment of children and women. Commercial surrogate motherhood might seem like the purchase of a baby, it might in some respect be like it, but it is not the purchase of a baby. Commercial surrogate motherhood is, perhaps, even more like the purchase of parenthood but it is not that either. One's love, say, might be ever so much like a red, red rose but it is not, thereby, a rose of whatever colour.

Anderson objects to C.S.M. and wants C.S.M. contracts not to be enforceable, because of the love that parents properly have for their children. She then adds:

'One might ask why this argument does not extend to all cases in which one might form an emotional attachment to an object one has contracted to sell. If I sign a contract with you to sell you my car, can I back out if I decide I am too emotionally attached to it? My argument is based upon the distinctive character of parental love, a mode of evaluation that should not be confused with less profound modes of evaluation that generate sentimental attachment to things. The degree to which other modes of valuation generate claims to consideration that tell against market norms remains an open question.' (Anderson, 1993, footnote 8: 229)

One is not and should not be allowed to buy and sell children – not because of how we feel about children but – because of what children are. If some particular parents do not have the sort of love of which Anderson speaks, it does not follow that they should be allowed to sell their children. If there were an entire generation of parents in some society none of whom had feelings of parental love, it would not be all right for babies to be sold in that society. It is the nature of children not the nature of parents, parental love or parenthood that renders the sale of babies morally wrong.

One is not and should not be allowed to buy and sell children. However, since C.S.M. is not the buying and selling of children, Anderson's comment is beside the point. Notice how the buying (or receiving the gift of) a car is quite different from becoming the parent of a child, no matter how one acquires the child. The rights and duties which parents have concerning their children differ considerably from those concerning their automobiles. Notice too that if one does contract to sell one's car and then, for whatever reason, changes one's mind, one might refuse to go through with the deal although not always with impunity nor without consequences. Even although the contract to sell the car was a legal one, it does not follow that one will be physically forced to part with it.

We take the view (and it is a 'norm' and 'value' of British society) -not that all actions should be legal or that all goods and services should be legally available for sale on the market but – that actions should be legal unless a good reason can be given for making them illegal and, similarly, that goods and services should be legally buyable and saleable unless a good reason can be given for making the buying and selling of them illegal. The onus is not on us to show that commercial surrogate motherhood agreements and commercial surrogate motherhood agencies should be legal. Rather, the onus is on those who want to make such transactions and agencies illegal to prove their case. That case is not established by the arguments that C.S.M. involves the commodification of babies and surrogate mothers and/or their services: either the commodification does not occur or, if it does occur, its occurrence is innocuous.

We are not proselytisers for C.S.M. We are not trying to encourage the practice nor to argue that more commercial surrogate motherhood is better than less. No: we are saying that if C.S.M. is to be legally restricted then this restriction requires a justification and that the arguments of Anderson and of Brazier *et al.* concerning commodification do not constitute such a justification.

It could turn out that there are good reasons for making C.S.M. illegal. Brazier *et al.* talk as if the only relevant interests concerned here were those of the parties directly concerned. They go further and talk of: '... the moral imperative to make the welfare of the child our prime concern' (p. 36). We think that the proper target of public policy lies elsewhere. For instance, if it could be shown that children born by commercial surrogate mothers are particularly delinquent and, throughout their adult lives, a burden to the other members of their communities and societies, then there might well be at least the basis of a powerful case for illegalising C.S.M.

The Brazier Report cannot be relied upon as a sound foundation for the formulation of wise public policies about surrogate motherhood. The remit of Brazier *et al.* was to consider whether, and if so, on what basis payments to surrogate mothers should be legal. They were told to consider this issue on the assumption that'... surrogacy should not be commercialised' (Brazier *et al.* p. 1). This assumption itself needs to be examined. The whole issue of surrogate motherhood and of commercial surrogate motherhood should be re-thought. Even more, perhaps, than this is required. The legacy for British public policy makers of the Brazier Report might be the unintended demonstration of the need for a radical re-assessment of the nature and proper scope of pecuniary transactions in connection with the provision of health care and related services (see for instance, Daar, 1998; Land and Dossetor, 1991; McLachlan, 1998 and 1999; Resnik, 1998; Thornton, 1999).

*By Hugh V McLachlan and J. Kim Swales from *Health Care Analysis*, 2000, Vol. 8, No. 1, pp. 1-18. With kind permission of Springer Sciences and Business Media.

Notes

(1) See Brazier *et al.*, 1998.
(2) See McLachlan, 1997a.
(3) Notice here that money, like all sources and forms of power can, in some respects, increase our autonomy just as poverty can reduce it. A surrogate mother, like other people, will have, in some respects, more autonomy when she has more rather than less money.
(40See McLachlan, 1997b.

References

Anderson, E. (1993) *Value in Ethics and Economics.* Harvard University Press: The MIT Press, Cambridge, MA.

Arneson, R. (1992) Commodification and Commercial Surrogacy. *Philosophy and Public Affairs 21,* 132-164.

Brazier, M., Campbell, A. and Golombok, S. (1998) *Surrogacy: Review for Health Ministers of Current Arrangements for Payments and Regulations;* Report of the Review Team, Cm 4068.

Daar, A.S. (1998) Paid Organ Donation – The Grey Basket Concept. *Journal of Medical Ethics* 24, 365-368.

Kornegay, R.J. (1990) Is Commercial Surrogacy Baby Selling? *Journal*

of Applied Philosophy 7, 45-50.
Land, W. and Dossetor, J.B. (Eds.) (1991) *Organ Replacement Therapy: Ethics, Justice and Commerce.* Berlin: Springer-Verlag.
McLachlan, H.V. (1997a) Bodies, Rights and Abortion. *Journal of Medical Ethics* 23, 176-180.
McLachlan, H.V. (1997b) Defending Commercial Surrogate Motherhood Against Van Niekerk and Van Zyl. *Journal of Medical Ethics* 23, 344-348.
McLachlan, H.V. (1998) The Un-Paid Donation of Blood and Altruism: A Comment on Keown. *Journal of Medical Ethics* 24, 252-254.
McLachlan, H.V. (1999) Altruism, Blood Donation and Public Policy: A Reply to Keown. *Journal of Medical Ethics,* Vol. 25, No.6.
McLachlan, H.V. and Swales, J.K. (1998) Commercial Surrogate Motherhood. *Contemporary Review,* 113-117.
Resnik, D. (1998) The Commodification of Human Reproductive Materials. *Journal of Medical Ethics* 24, 388-393.
Thornton, J. (1999) *Should Health Screening be Private?* The I.E.A. Health and Welfare Unit, Choice in Welfare No. 48.
van Niekerk, A. and van Zyl, L. (1995a) Commercial Surrogacy and the Commodification of Children: An Ethical Perspective. *Medicine and Law* 14, 163-170.
van Niekerk, A. and van Zyl, L. (1995b) The Ethics of Surrogacy: Women's Reproductive Labour. *Journal of Medical Ethics* 21, 345-349.
Werthheimer, A. (1996) *Exploitation.* Princeton: Princeton University Press.

Chapter Eleven

Scotland, the Church and Surrogate Motherhood*

Introduction

Public policy measures concerning surrogate motherhood and, in particular, commercial surrogate motherhood have been suggested recently by the Brazier Report (1998) and by a Study Group of the Church of Scotland (1996). We shall discuss them and their suggested *rationale*. It is our intention to draw attention to this debate and to suggest that the issues have as yet been insufficiently debated; our aim is not to give an exhaustive, definitive or convincingly conclusive account of it. The debate remains an open one.

The continuation of this debate would be interesting and important, we suggest, under any circumstances, but particularly so given the existence of the Scottish Parliament and the swelling appearance of a Scottish political identity. Not only is there now a locus in Scotland for customised discussions of and decisions about such a social and moral issue as surrogate motherhood but the contributions from Scotland to UK-wide (and wider) political debates – about, for instance, surrogate motherhood – might have an even more distinctive Scottish flavour and focus than they have had hitherto.

We shall focus in this paper particularly – but not exclusively – on what is called 'gestational surrogate motherhood', what might be thought of as the 'purest' sort of surrogate motherhood. This is where a couple are the genetic parents of a child which, say, through a deformity of the womb, the woman is unable to carry and bear for herself and another women – a substitute mother or, to use the synonym which is invariably employed, a 'surrogate' mother -carries it in her stead.

Here is the position from which we approach the issue. We are not antagonistic to the Church of Scotland: indeed, one of us is a member of it. We are not enthusiasts for commercial surrogate motherhood or for surrogate motherhood. We do not think that the world would necessarily be a better place for more rather than less of it. We have no interest in promoting it nor desire to promote it. However, we take the view that surrogate motherhood and commercial surrogate motherhood and commercial surrogate motherhood agencies – just like any other activities – should be legal unless their illegality can be justified. The onus is on those who would ban to justify any suggested ban. We are not in any sense uncritical 'free-marketeers'. (See McLachlan 1994.) Not everything should be legally available for sale on a market. Markets should (and always do) operate within a context of legal regulation. Legal restrictions can, of course, be justified. They should be justified, we suggest, or removed.

Father Tom Connelly, the Roman Catholic Church's Press Officer in Scotland is quoted, in *The Herald*, as challenging views on commercial surrogate motherhood which we expressed (or were thought to express) in a conference paper[2]. He says: '… first of all a child is not a product, and while everyone has sympathy for childless couples, nobody has a right to a child' (Smith 1998, p. 10). We agree with this entirely. Some people, when they defend surrogate motherhood, might do so on the suggested grounds that people have a 'right' to be parents: we do not. When people are conceived and born, they are not conceived and born of right but of supreme good fortune. Similarly those by whom they are conceived do not conceive them of right. It does not follow from this that surrogate motherhood is wrong nor that it should be illegal.

Surrogate Motherhood: The Current Legal Position

The relevant legislation concerning surrogate motherhood in the UK is the Surrogacy Arrangements Act 1985 and section 30 of the Human Fertilisation and Embryology Act 1990.

It is not a criminal offence for a commissioning couple to pay a surrogate mother for carrying a child: however, such agreements – along with all surrogate motherhood agreements, whether commercial or not – are not legally enforceable. Moreover, when a commissioning couple make an application to the courts to be recognised as the legal parents of the child in question (either through adoption or by the granting of a parental order) their application could be refused if they have made, unless authorised by the court to do so, payment in excess of reasonable expenses to a surrogate mother. Nonetheless, in practice, the courts have tended not to deny legal parenthood on this basis: rather, they have retrospectively authorised the payments at whatever level they have happened to be.

It can be a crime to act in an entrepreneurial capacity in relation to surrogate motherhood. As Brazier *et al.* note: '… section 2 of the Surrogacy Arrangements Act 1985 prohibited any person from assisting in the making of a surrogacy arrangement on a commercial basis, thus preventing commercial "agencies" from operating to assist in the creation of surrogacy arrangements' (1998, p 24). It is not clear

– or, at least, it is not clear to us – whether the objection of the law makers is to the assisting in – whether for payment or not – a commercial arrangement between a commissioning couple and a surrogate mother or to the paid assisting in a surrogate arrangement, whether or not it is a commercial one. Notice that various people, for instance, doctors, lawyers and counsellors, will receive fees – and fees well in excess of expenses reasonably incurred – from commissioning couples in return for services provided for them in relation to surrogate motherhood. As Brazier *et al.* say: '... several professionals may be involved in the consequences of surrogacy arrangements. All are likely to be paid by the commissioning couple and may perceive their primary interest as being to that couple' (p.24). Whether or not such activities are, technically, crimes, the law is not interested in pursuing them. Instead, it is the actions of those agents (and agencies) who (and which), for a fee, help commissioning parents and surrogate mothers who want to meet to meet which run foul of the law and to which it is not likely to be blind.

Notice that the commissioning couple might pay a surrogate mother for the carrying of a child and not receive the child. The couple would be unable to sue in a court for the return of the money. Similarly, a surrogate mother might, in return for promised money, carry a child, give it to the commissioning parents and fail to receive the money. She too would have no legal redress. However, if the parents or surrogate mother refused to pay a doctor, lawyer or counsellor for services rendered in connection with these deals which were reneged on, one suspects that they could and would be sued – and rightly so – by the professional people in question.

It is against the law to advertise either the services of or the desire for the services of a carrying mother. Notwithstanding, there are at least two non-commercial surrogate motherhood agencies in Britain and they operate quite openly and legally, they are Childlessness Overcome Through Surrogacy and the Surrogate Parenting Centre.

The Brazier Report

In June 1997, partly, at least, because there was in some minds disquiet about the existence of 'commercial' surrogate motherhood and of payments to surrogate mothers in excess of 'reasonable expenses', the UK Health Ministers asked Professor Brazier, Professor Campbell and Professor Golombok to review certain aspects of the current law and practice concerning surrogate motherhood. (This trio is, respectively, a lawyer, an ethicist and a psychologist.)

The remit of the Brazier Review Team was to consider the possibility and desirability of regulating surrogate motherhood arrangements and in particular to consider whether payments of any sort to the surrogate mother should be legal. It was a specification of the remit 'that surrogacy should not be commercialised and that any woman who has a baby as part of a surrogacy arrangement should not be compelled to give it up if she changes her mind' (p. 1).

The Brazier Report (1998) recommended that surrogate mothers should be paid, by commissioning parents, only in regard to actual expenses caused by the pregnancy. It recommended the continuation of section 1A of the 1985 Surrogacy Act whereby the non-enforceability of surrogate motherhood contracts (and not merely commercial ones) was iterated. It recommended that only 'non-profit making' surrogate motherhood agencies should be legally allowed and that they should be registered with the UK Departments of Health.

In the report, it is written:

We recommend the enactment of a new Surrogacy Act to ban payments other than expenses, to require the registration of surrogacy agencies and to give statutory force to a Code of Practice. Contraventions of the ban on payments to the surrogate [mother] other than expenses would result in ineligibility for a parental order. It would become a criminal offence to operate an unregistered surrogacy agency. (Brazier *et al.* 1998, p. ii)

With regard to the reasons for these recommendations, the report says:

'We find that payments to surrogate mothers, other than in recompense for genuine expenses, give rise to the following concerns. (1) Payments create a danger that women will give less than free and fully informed consent to act as a surrogate [mother]. (2) Payments risk the commodification of the child to be born. (3) Payments contravene the social norms of our society that, just as bodily parts cannot be sold, nor can such intimate services'. (Brazier *et al.* 1998, p. i)

We shall return to (2) when we consider the claims made in the Report of the Church of Scotland Study Group. Prior to that, we shall comment briefly on arguments (1) and (3).

Brazier and her colleagues were concerned, in relation to (1), that, typically, surrogate mothers are poorer and less educated than the commissioning parents with whom they deal and that, consequently, commercial surrogate arrangements are likely to be exploitative of the surrogate mothers. If this is a warranted concern, then it might be thought to be even more relevant in the Scottish context than in that of the UK in general given that the per capita income in Scotland is lower than in the UK: there might be the worry that, typically, English commissioning parents will exploit Scottish surrogate mothers[3]. However, it is far from clear first of all that commercial surrogate motherhood is exploitative and secondly that, if it is, the Brazier recommendations are justified.

Perhaps it is unfair that some people are poorer and less educated than others but it does not follow that any transaction with them is necessarily unfair or exploitative. There is a difference between driving someone to the wall and transacting – perhaps fairly and non-exploitatively – with someone who is already at the wall (Wertheimer 1996). There is a distinction too between saying that something is exploitative and showing that, because it is exploitative, it should be illegal or otherwise discouraged by public policies. For instance, Marxists, after all, think that, within capitalism, the relationship between employers and employees is 'exploitative' but not necessarily that employment, within capitalism, should be illegal or be discouraged by public policy. There are worse things than being 'exploited': being saved from 'exploitation' can sometimes be one of them.

Paternalistic intervention, which is what argument (1) calls for, is sometimes justified but it is justified, when it is, only if the paternalists actually do know better than the people who are being treated paternalistically what the best interests of the latter are. There seems no reason to assume that this condition is met in this case. If potential surrogate mothers – whether or not they are wealthy and well educated – want to be surrogate mothers, are willing to run the risks involved and want to accept money for the services they provide and they disagree with Brazier and her colleagues when the latter say that such actions are not in their best interests then, to say the least, it is far from clear on what basis one could say that Brazier and her colleagues are more likely than the potential surrogate mothers to be right.

Argument (3) is related to the notion that it is good to donate body parts and services but bad to sell them, and that gift relationships are invariably better than commercial ones. Perhaps, if it is true as is often supposed that Scottish people in general are more 'left wing' and less pro-capitalist than are people in general in the UK, then the 'social norms' which Brazier and her colleagues talk about might be particularly powerful in Scotland. However, this would only mean that (3) might be a popular argument in Scotland, not that it would be a sound one.

Furthermore, it is not clear that (3) is actually an argument at all rather than the mere assertion that a particular point of view is commonly held. What is wrong with selling bodily parts and services? What is the argument against it? In any event, it is not the case that the selling of all bodily parts is illegal. Human sperm, for instance, can, legally, be bought and sold. It is not clear that this state of affairs causes any general feeling – whether appropriate or not – of outrage. It might be argued that services which are just as 'intimate' as the services of a carrying mother can be and commonly are legally bought and sold. There will be different views about what counts as 'intimacy' – what about the services of, say, a dentist, a chiropodist, a gynaecologist, a geriatric nurse or an artist's model? What a carrying mother does for the carried baby might be an 'intimate' service. That which she does for the commissioning parents, some might think, is not.

The Church of Scotland

Pre-Conceived Ideas: A Christian Perspective of IVF and Embryology (Church of Scotland 1996) is the Report of the Study Group on Human Fertilisation and Embryology, which was produced by the Board of Social Responsibility of the Church of Scotland. The Study Group is very opposed to surrogate motherhood, particularly, but not only, commercial surrogate motherhood. Its public policy recommendations are not as fully specified as those of the Brazier report but it is clear that they are as restrictive as, and perhaps even more restrictive than, those of the latter (and later) publication. Summarising the position taken by the Church of Scotland (and, apparently, still held) and expressed previously in Reports in 1982 and 1985, they say: '… surrogacy should be made illegal' (Church of Scotland 1996, p.5). However, they do not further specify what form this illegality should take or what should be its consequences.

Writing in 1996 and talking about the then current situation, they say: '… the Study Group is aware that the law in the UK is designed to discourage surrogacy without criminalising the families directly involved. It would not want to see the law liberalised' (Church of Scotland 1996, p. 78). Would the Church of Scotland want the law – in Scotland?; in the UK?; in both?; everywhere? – to be less liberal than that proposed by the Brazier Report? Would it agree entirely with the Brazier Report's recommendations? It would be fascinating to know. Our hunch is that the Brazier recommendations would be 'too liberal' for the Church of Scotland or, more specifically, for its Study Group.

The opposition to surrogate motherhood of the Study Group is said by them to be based on the following reasons:

- '... it is an intrusion into the marriage relationship and undermines the divinely ordained bond of husband, wife, and child within the family' (Church of Scotland 1996, p.78).
- '... it requires of the surrogate mother a detachment which in other circumstances one would not look for in a mother. A willingness to give up her child, which in an ordinary mother would be seen as a fault, becomes a virtue in a surrogate mother. The physical, psychological and spiritual bonding between mother and child which is an important part of pregnancy is denied' (Church of Scotland 1996, pp.78-79).
- '... where surrogacy is a commercial arrangement, the dignity of the child is violated through its becoming an object of barter' (Church of Scotland 1996, p.79).

Let us consider each of these arguments of the Church of Scotland in turn.

Incompatibility with the Christian Concept of Marriage

It is useful to couple the first objection of the Church of Scotland to surrogate motherhood with the claim of theirs that surrogacy is '... incompatible with the Christian concept of marriage' (p.5). Now, there are two general replies which we would make in response to this objection. First of all, that something is not ordained by God or is not in accordance with the Christian concept of, say, marriage, is in itself no good reason for making it a crime. (Did God ordain that those actions which were not in accordance with His will should be crimes? If so, where and how did He make this ordinance manifest?) Secondly, it is far from clear that surrogate motherhood is against the will of God or at variance with the concept (or concepts?) of Christian marriage. Where, for instance, can Christ be cited as having spoken against surrogate motherhood?

The Church of Scotland accepts the Ten Commandments and believes that it is ordained by God that people should, for instance, honour God, honour their father and mother, remember the Sabbath day to keep it holy, and refrain from committing adultery. It would be alarming to hear, particularly given the existence of the

Scottish Parliament, that it is the view of the Church of Scotland that such breaches of the Commandments should be made into crimes.

Often, even when particular actions are in themselves immoral, it is wise not to make them crimes. Whether something is morally wrong (or sinful) and whether it would be a good idea to make it illegal are quite distinct questions. Adultery, for instance, is or can be a wrong and highly immoral action. Many religious people, including members of the Church of Scotland, would consider it to be sinful. In some countries adultery is a crime. In Scotland, adultery was once a crime. Indeed, it was once a capital offence (McLachlan and Swales 1993). It does not follow that if adultery is immoral or a sin it should be made criminal. Does the Church of Scotland want adultery in Scotland to be again a crime on the grounds that it is incompatible with Christian marriage and: '... is an intrusion into the marriage relationship and undermines the divinely ordained bond of husband, wife, and child within the family'? (p.78). One assumes that it does not, even although adultery, manifestly, causes more problems and unhappiness than the less widespread practice of surrogate motherhood is every likely to do.

It would seem to be immoral and highly un-Christian for Christians to accuse other people of un-Christian behaviour unless they have extremely strong grounds for claiming that the behaviour in question is un-Christian. A problem here is that no Biblical sources are quoted by the Study Group in support of their view that surrogate motherhood is un-Christian. In *Genesis*, Chapter 16, a situation is narrated which is, or is like, surrogate motherhood[4]. Sarai, the wife of Abram, is barren and, at her suggestion, he fathers a child -who was called Ishmael – of Hagar, her handmaid. The arrangement is not condemned in the Bible. No reference is made to this portion of the Scriptures or to any other one.

A corollary of the doctrine of the virgin birth is that Joseph, the husband of Mary and the social father of Jesus was not His biological father. Given this, it is not easy to see how it can be justifiably argued that there is one and only one acceptable form of Christian family unit. Even if one were to ignore the doctrine of the virgin birth, it is difficult to see how one could justifiably argue that there is one and only one acceptable form of Christian family unit. What could be the theological objection to, say, fostering or adoption? Should they, on theological grounds, be made criminal?

It is unconvincing to say that a gestational surrogate mother 'undermines the divinely ordained bond of husband, wife, and child within the family' since, in the sort of cases we are talking about, without her, there could be no bond between the child and the husband and wife since the child is dependent upon the surrogate mother for the chance of existence. The child would not be born were it not for the help of the surrogate mother.

If a husband and wife need and seek the assistance of, say, a sex psychotherapist, a gynaecologist, and a midwife in order to assist them to have a baby, would one say that such people are an intrusion into their marriage? It would be strange to do so. Similarly, if it is the case that a husband and wife can have what is genetically their own baby only if a surrogate mother carries the embryo, fetus and baby for them and if they request someone to perform that service for them, it is very odd to condemn the service or the person providing it as necessarily being an 'intrusion' into the marriage.

Surrogate Motherhood is Different

The second objection of the Church of Scotland might be true. However, it does not seem to be relevant. Three points are being made here and with the first two of them we agree without reservation. About the third one we are sceptical. However, these points (even if true) do not serve to show that surrogacy is wrong, merely that it is different and that, in fact, surrogate motherhood is surrogate motherhood. A description of surrogate motherhood is not in itself a criticism of it far less a reason for making it illegal.

It is true that surrogate mothers are expected to act in ways which would be condemnable in normal mothers but surrogate mothers are not normal mothers. Consider, for instance, foster parents. They too are expected to act, in some circumstances, in ways in which one would not expect or want normal parents to act. Foster parents, for instance, are sometimes required to sever links with children whom they have grown to love and who have grown to love and depend on them. What would be a fault in a normal mother or father can be a virtue in a foster parent. Foster mothers, like surrogate mothers are not normal mothers but neither surrogate motherhood or fostering are condemnable merely on that account.

Surrogate motherhood is not ideal; it is resorted to only because the ideal is not available to the couple concerned. It would bizarre to say that children should not be born at all – and surrogate motherhood is, we are assuming, the only possible basis for the birth of these particular children – if the children cannot be bonded with their parents in the normal way. Such children, the Church of Scotland seems here to suggest, should be denied everything, should not be allowed to live, because their genetic mothers are incapable of providing them with a normal pregnancy.

More thought should be given by the Study Group to their argument here. Perhaps they mean something other than what they are or seem to be saying.

Commercial Surrogate Motherhood and the Dignity of the Child

This is very similar to the contention of Brazier *et al.* that: 'payments risk the commodification of the child to be born'. It is similar too to a claim made in response to our views on surrogate motherhood by Father Tom Connelly that: 'it is wrong even when money doesn't enter into it. And when it does, then we have trafficking in human life' (Smith 1998, p. 10).

Now, even if this objection of the Church of Scotland were true, it would not be a devastating criticism of surrogate and commercial surrogate motherhood. After all, it is surely better to be born with one's dignity violated than not to be born at all. If the only way that a particular person could be born is through becoming an object of barter then no obvious favour is being done to that person by failing to allow him to become an object of barter.

However, it is not true that, with commercial surrogate motherhood, children are objects of 'barter': neither are children 'commodities' or, necessarily, thereby treated as 'commodities' or as mere objects. Notice the inappropriate, emotive and loaded use of the word 'barter' here. 'Barter' is the wrong word to use. Barter, which is typically a form of economic exchange, involves trading objects and commodities for objects and commodities rather than for money. Commercial surrogate motherhood usually involves a monetary exchange. Similarly, the word 'traffic', used by Father Connelly, is a gratuitously pejorative one, connoting a trade in that which should not be traded.

Commercial surrogate motherhood is not the buying or selling of babies. Babies are not owned by anyone. They are not possible objects of purchase or sale (under, Scottish, English and all other legal systems of which we are aware). Similarly, the legal rights of parenthood, which, in a sense, is what commissioning parents in a surrogacy arrangement want to have, are not purchasable either. Neither the gestational mother or the genetic mother owns the baby or the child. The question of one or other of them buying or selling it does not arise. The gestational mother, under English and Scots law, would normally be assumed to be the legal mother of the child. The commissioning couple, the genetic mother and father of the child in this case, could apply to the courts for a parental rights order and they would hope that the gestational mother would not pursue – that she would waive – her legal rights concerning the child. It is wrong to say that commercial surrogate motherhood involves buying a baby. If you buy, say, a house or a motor car, then you have legal rights and duties concerning that motor car which others do not have. If you 'buy' a baby, what rights and duties do you have which differ from those which parents have towards their children who were born in the normal way? None. Children acquired as a result of commercial surrogate motherhood do not became nor are they necessarily treated as 'objects' or 'commodities'.

What is bought and sold with commercial surrogate motherhood is the services of the carrying mother (and, sometimes the entrepreneurial and related services of commercial surrogate motherhood agencies and agents). One could say too that the payment might induce the carrying mother to promise not to pursue her legal rights of parenthood concerning the child. This is not quite the same as saying that she sells her legal rights nor that the commissioning parent purchase legal rights. As in any transaction, what people actually buy; what they think they are buying; what they expect to receive; and what they will receive can be four separate matters. This is one of the reasons why, in general, laws and legal processes are useful and why, in particular, there is a strong case for making commercial surrogate motherhood contracts legal and legally enforceable.

If you pay a taxi driver to convey your body and your baby's body from one place to another or, as you might do in some cultures and circumstances, if you pay a porter to carry you or your baby from one place to another, you are not thereby involved in some sort of immoral action. You are not treating the taxi driver or the porter or your own body or your baby's body as a mere object or a mere commodity. Similarly, if a couple give a fertilised egg of theirs to a surrogate mother and pay her for carrying it, delivering it as a baby and returning to them in that form, they do not seem to be treating the baby as a mere commodity. They do not seem, in any way which is wrong, to be 'trafficking in human life'. They do not seem to be violating the dignity of the child concerned: rather, what they are doing in the context represents an appropriate manifestation of love and respect towards the child. They are certainly not buying a baby – their own biological baby – from the surrogate mother. After all, and the analogy is incomplete, if you pay a haulier to carry a trunk for you from, say, Glasgow to Leeds, and, at the handing over of money in Leeds, the trunk is returned to you, you would not consider that you were buying the trunk from the haulier.

If this particular objection, relating to 'dignity' and 'barter' of the Study Group to commercial surrogate motherhood has any relevant force, then some work is required by them to show what it is.

Conclusion

In the case of both the Brazier Report and the Report of the Church of Scotland, there is a gulf between their recommendations and the arguments which they put forward to support them.

The recommendations concerning the legalisation of commercial surrogate motherhood agencies are, in our view, particularly unconvincing. The hostility of Brazier and her colleagues to them is inexplicable. Organisations such as, for instance, universities, churches and matrimonial agencies -whether or not they are all 'commercial' or 'profit-making' (whatever, precisely such terms mean or signify) – are allowed to advertise their services; they are allowed to charge fees; people such as Professor Brazier and us and ministers and priests can, legally, make a living from working for them. Even in terms of the *rationale* of the Brazier report, it is unclear why commercial surrogate motherhood agencies should be treated so differently from them. It is unclear too why surrogate motherhood agencies should be registered with ministries of health. The particular services which they provide are no more, in themselves, health services than are, say, the services provided by matrimonial agencies or singles bars. The particular services which they provide are hardly likely to be more efficiently provided by virtue of such registration. Why, too, should commissioning couples not be allowed, at the very least, to pay to such agencies and agents 'reasonable expenses'?

It is not clear why or that it would be unwise to allow such agencies to operate as straight-forward 'profit-making' and 'commercial' ones. In the Brazier Report, it is said of the organisation Childlessness Overcome Through Surrogacy that: '… their preferred solution is a regulated commercial market' (Brazier *et al.* 1998, p. 25). We would say that this is the solution which should be adopted unless a justification can be given for deviating from it. Childlessness

Overcome Through Surrogacy are not required to prove to people who disagree with them that commercial surrogate motherhood should be legal. Rather, the onus of proof is on those who advocate the illegality of commercial surrogate motherhood – a burden which the writers of neither of the reports we have looked at have, so far, managed to discharge.

If a gestational surrogate mother does not want to return a child which she has carried to the genetic parents, what should be done? This might well be a very difficult legal and moral question. It is not obvious that the wishes of the carrying mother should always trump those of the genetic parents if she wants to go back on her word. There is, perhaps, more of a dilemma here than a problem with a solution or a question with an answer. However, it is far from clear that the difficulties will be lessened, far less removed, by the non-enforceability of surrogate motherhood contracts. 'Enforceability', after all, might be limited to the granting of compensation for breaches of contract. 'Enforceability' need not mean the forced removal of a child from a surrogate mother. Whether, on some occasions at least, it should mean that is another issue, which the non-enforceability of surrogate motherhood contracts evades rather than solves.

Perhaps the recommendations which Brazier and the Church of Scotland Study Group make could be sustained by arguments other than those which they put forward. Perhaps the acceptance of alternative recommendations concerning surrogate motherhood and commercial surrogate motherhood would be preferable. In either case, the debate concerning surrogate motherhood requires continuation. We should say, perhaps, that the debates require continuation since the Scottish Parliament and the UK Parliament might, in the end, settle on different policy measures and different legislation concerning surrogate motherhood with all the interesting complications which that might produce.

*By Hugh V. McLachlan and J.K. Swales from *Scottish Affairs*, no.32, summer 2000, pp. 111-123.

Notes

(1) From the evidence of the limited sample considered by Brazier (1998), it would appear that around a quarter (24%) of surrogate mothers are gestational surrogate mothers.

(2) The conference was the Scottish Economic Society's Annual

Conference, held at Glasgow Caledonian University, 7-8th April 1998. The paper we gave was entitled: 'Babies, Child Bearers and Commodities: The Political Economy of Commercial Surrogate Motherhood'. See Smith (1998) and Stewart (1998).

(3) Note that Brazier gives no evidence to suggest that, typically, surrogate mothers are poorer and less well educated than are commissioning parents. Perhaps the assumption is false. According to a study which we came across on the Internet: 'In contrast to the stereotype of a heartless, misguided impoverished woman primarily motivated by money, surrogates emerge here as average mothers, often trying to further the goals of their children and families' (Aigen 1996).

(4) We are grateful to Lynne Craig, a 4th Year Social Sciences student at Glasgow Caledonian University, for drawing this passage to our attention.

References

Aigen, Betsey P. (1996), 'Motivations of Surrogate Mothers: Parenthood, Altruism and Self-Actualization' TASC@surrogacy.com.

Brazier, Margaret (1998), *Surrogacy: Review for Health Ministers of Current Arrangement for Payments and Regulation; Report of the Review Team*, The Stationery Office, Cm 4068.

Church of Scotland (1996), *Pre-Conceived Ideas: A Christian Perspective of IVF and Embryology*, Church of Scotland, Study Group on Human Fertilisation and Embryology, Si. Andrews Press, Edinburgh.

McLachlan, Hugh V. (1985), 'In Defence of Surrogate Motherhood', *Contemporary Review*, January.

McLachlan, Hugh V. (1994), 'Freedom and the Market: A Defence of 'Socialist' Intervention', *The Philosopher*, Autumn.

McLachlan, Hugh V. (1997), 'Defending Commercial Surrogate Motherhood Against Van Nierkerk and Van Zyl', *Journal of Medical Ethics*, Vol. 23, No. 6.

McLachlan, Hugh V. and Swales, J.K. (1998), 'Commercial Surrogate Motherhood', *Contemporary Review*, March.

McLachlan, Hugh V. and Swales, J.K. (1993), 'Sexual Bias and the Law: The Case of Pre-Industrial Scotland', *International Journal of Sociology and Social Policy*, Vol. 14, No. 9 1993.

McLachlan, Hugh V. and Swales, J.K. (1997), 'Provider of Service Worthy of Payment', *The Scotsman*, 12th June, p. 6.

Smith, Ken (1998), 'Surrogacy for cash defended', *The Herald*, 9th,

April, p. 10.
Stewart, Graeme (1998), 'Commercial surrogacy not immoral, say academics', *The Scotsman*, 8th April, p. 10.
Wertheimer, Alan (1996), *Exploitation*, Princeton University Press, Princeton, New Jersey.

Chapter Twelve

Exploitation and Commercial Surrogate Motherhood*

Introduction

Various authors have argued that commercial surrogate motherhood (C.S.M.) is exploitative and, because of its claimed exploitative nature, it should be prohibited. Here, we examine their arguments and conclude that they are not compelling.

The term 'exploitation' is one that is often used without sufficient clarity and care, as Wertheimer convincingly argues (See Wertheimer, 1996). It is often used as a general term of disapproval, where the user gives the false impression that a specific analytic meaning is attached to it. Wertheimer talks of exploitation in relation to actions and relationships but it is mainly transactions that interest him. The kernel of his account is that a transaction between A and B is exploitative when A takes an unfair advantage of B. He distinguishes between this and the taking by A of an advantage of an unfairness which might exist in B's situation. There is, as he shows, an important although often neglected difference between (fairly or unfairly) pushing someone to the wall and dealing (fairly or unfairly) with someone who is already at the wall.

According to Levine: 'Exploitation refers to our use of others as means to our ends, often ends involving acquisition of wealth, without due regard for their personhood. By using others in this way, we debase them as persons. To exploit someone is wrongfully to claim the product of his or her labor, talent, ingenuity' (Levine, 1997,p.87). Levine suggests that this 'wrongfulness' is related to some idea of 'justice'. This coheres with what Scruton says in his claim that: 'In common parlance, John exploits Alfred when John uses Alfred to John's advantage and Alfred's detriment without making just recompense (perhaps making no recompense whatever). Hence application of the idea of exploitation presupposes a standard of "just recompense"' (Scruton, 1982, p. 162). Here, what is interesting is that 'exploitation' may be considered as an unjust treatment or even a particular sort of unjust treatment. Maybe it is a violation of another's right of recipience particularly regarding monetary amounts (See McLachlan, 1998). If justice and fairness are different notions, this is similar but not identical to Wertheimer's account of exploitation.

Unequal bargaining power can be a cause of exploitation but it is not the only possible cause. The exercise of unequal bargaining power is not inevitably or inherently exploitative. Obviously, states are far more powerful than individual citizens but states do not invariably or inevitably exploit their citizens: they often treat them justly. Some citizens, through, for example, tax evasion defraud the state. Thus, the less powerful can exploit the more powerful.

Let us imagine that a highwayman who, far richer than a particular passenger in a stage-coach, persuades her to part with her necklace by offering money for it. The passenger is not necessarily being exploited. If she is persuaded to part with it by the threat of a broken head, she is being exploited no matter how rich or powerful the highwayman or the passenger may be.

Exploitation, then, is more involved with strategies – with unfair and/or unjust strategies – than with the exercise of power as such (See Hindess, 1982). In this regard, the breach of norms, conventions and laws is often relevant. So, too, is the use and misuse of information. Cheating at cards would be an example of exploitation even though achieving the same outcome through, for example, an abnormally powerful memory would not. The issue of the division of the spoils is also relevant to the notion of exploitation. If the passenger was forced by the highwayman – by the threat of a broken head – into a transaction with the highwayman, then the passenger would have emerged worse off than she would have been had the transaction not occurred and had the 'offer' of the transaction not been made. Of the benefits of the transaction, all were directed to the highwayman.

Of course, this is an extreme case. In some circumstances, where both parties benefit from a transaction, the transaction might be thought to be exploitative because of the unfair and disproportionately large benefits accruing to one of the parties, at the expense of the other. Notice that 'exploitation' is not always used in a pejorative sense. For instance, one might talk with approval of the exploitation of, for example, natural resources or technology.

Anderson, Commercial Surrogate Motherhood, Exploitation and Fraud

Anderson claims that C.S.M. is immoral and should be illegal because it involves exploitation and fraud, but her reasons for so claiming are neither clear nor convincing[1]. Her claims provoke this initial reaction. If the surrogate mother receives a sufficiently high fee, then one could consider that the fear relating to exploitation would be groundless. If, no matter how high the fee is, the surrogate mother is, somehow, still 'exploited', then one is brought to wonder what is so wrong with 'exploitation' as Anderson conceives it and to wonder why she wants to make it illegal. It might or might not be regrettable that some people are required to be, for example, university lectures, or surrogate mothers, or the employees of rich capitalists in order to acquire a livelihood but, given the existence of this requirement, the means of meeting it would, on the face of it, merit a welcome rather than an attack.

Anderson (1993, p. 186) responds to comments of this sort by suggesting that:

'...the significant forms of exploitation involved in contract pregnancy are emotional, not financial. It would be difficult to recruit suitable candidates for surrogate motherhood without engaging in fraudulent exploitation'.

She continues by stating that:

'It would be strange if I thought mothers were financially exploited in the parenting contract, since I hold that no one is entitled to profit financially from selling their children. Their exploitation is emotional and consists in the fact that the surrogate industry and its clients often raise emotional expectations they plan to frustrate once they have ceased to be useful' (1993, footnote 6, p.229).

Lies can be told and fraud (in the moral and legal senses) can occur with contracts and relationships of any sort but this is hardly a reason for making all relationships and all contracts illegal[2]. For instance, people can enter into marriage, as lying, deceitful, bigamists but this in itself is not a good reason for saying that marriage, as such, should be made illegal (although some particular marriages are and should be illegal). Similarly, some commercial surrogate agents and agencies might lie, be deceitful and/or engage in fraud. Presumably, such fraudulent commercial activity *qua* fraudulent commercial activity would be and should be illegal. There is no need to say that fraudulent commercial surrogacy should be illegal when fraud itself is illegal. What Anderson fails to demonstrate is that, by their very nature, all commercial surrogate motherhood contracts and the activities which are undertaken to try to secure them are inherently and inevitably fraudulent. Furthermore, one might suggest that if the problem resides in the lack of adequate useful information given to the surrogate mothers, then a solution could be found through the means of providing it for them.

That C.S.M. is inherently, as Anderson claims, 'emotional exploitation' is far from being demonstrated. What she means by 'emotional exploitation', remains mysterious. Moreover, whether or not it is emotionally exploitative, that C.S.M. should be illegal is not established by her. If, through the threat of a violent death, a highwayman convinces a woman to become a surrogate mother, then his action is 'exploitative' and is and should be illegal. If, on the other hand, he convinces a woman to become a surrogate mother by the offer of money, then, to say the least, it is very far from obvious that the action is exploitative and/or that it should be made illegal.

Tong, Commercial Surrogate Motherhood, Feminism and Exploitation

Tong indicates that some feminists state that when a women consents to be a commercial surrogate mother, such apparently 'free' choices are the product of economic coercion and that:

'These feminists note that most surrogate mothers, like most prostitutes, are much poorer than the people to whom they sell their services. Unable to get a decent job, a woman may be driven to sell her body if it is the only thing she has that anyone seems to value enough to buy. But to say that a woman "chooses" to do this, claim feminist opponents of surrogacy, is to say that when a woman is forced to choose between being poor and being exploited, she may choose being exploited as the lesser of two evils' (Tong, 1997, pp. 200-201).

If this is what exploitation is, why should exploitation be illegal? Why should the option of the lesser evil be denied to poor people? If relative poverty is wrong, then one should condemn that rather than the means of alleviating it. To concede that C.S.M. is 'exploitation' need not be to say that it should be made illegal. After all, Marxists might say that the proletariat are being 'exploited' when they are employed by capitalists without suggesting that, under capitalism, it should be made illegal for capitalists to employ members of the proletariat. Perhaps it would be better if the world were different so that no one would want nor need to work for a capitalist and no one would want nor need to be a commercial surrogate mother: but that is not the question at issue.

We agree with Wertheimer who suggests that:

'If a woman can reasonably regard surrogacy as improving her overall welfare given that society has unjustly limited her options, it is arguable that it would be adding insult to injury to deny her that opportunity. Whatever label we use to describe her choice, we must still decide whether she should be allowed to make such a choice' (1996, p.l 1).

Call it "exploitation" if you want; the question remains: should C.S.M. be legal or illegal? After all, not all "exploitation" is criminalised. However, it is not obvious that C.S.M. is necessarily "exploitation". We do not concede that it is exploitative. If voluntary commercial surrogate motherhood is said to be 'exploitative', then why not say that all employment when the employees would rather not have to be employees is exploitative? (See Wertheimer 1996, p. 109)

Here, we are inclined to the view that if there is exploitation, there must be an exploiter: one cannot be exploited by events and circumstances but only by agents and agencies. Events and circumstances, such as poverty, might make one vulnerable to being exploited and might make one susceptible to the temptation to lie and to cheat and be an exploiter but in neither case is the exploitation inevitable nor is it necessarily a feature of the situation. C.S.M., like employment in general, can be, but need not be, exploitative. For example, if a highwayman forces a traveller to make the choice: 'your money or your life', then the highwayman might be said to 'exploit' the traveller by stealing his/her money or, even worse, if he carries out his threat, by killing the traveller and stealing the money. The highwayman creates a 'need'. If the highwayman leaves the scene, the traveller does not need to part with his/her money in order to retain his/her life. This is quite unlike the case of commercial surrogate motherhood. Neither the surrogate motherhood agency nor the commissioning parents create the need to make a living for actual or potential surrogate mothers. They offer a means of meeting an already existing need. There is a difference between being 'forced' into a transaction with, for example, a butcher by hunger and being forced into a transaction with a butcher by the butcher. We would not – although others might – consider the former sort of transaction to be 'exploitation'. Similarly, if a woman is driven by economic need to choose to become a commercial surrogate mother, we would not consider this to be exploitation. The situation might be condemnable and regrettable on other grounds but that is another matter.

The Warnock Report

The Warnock Report, published in 1984 and re-published in Warnock (1985) recommended, among other things, that commercial surrogate motherhood agencies should be prohibited and that all surrogate motherhood contracts should be illegal and unenforceable.

This was done because the Warnock Report attacks C.S.M. as being 'exploitative'. Concerning surrogate motherhood, it states: 'That people should treat others as a means to their own ends, however desirable the consequences, must always be liable to moral objection. Such treatment of one person by another becomes positively exploitative when financial interests are involved' (Warnock, 1985, p.46). But if we go, for example, to a dentist for treatment to alleviate toothache, we treat the dentist – or his/her services – as a means to our own desired ends. Nothing in this situation, as described, is morally objectionable. Whatever Kant might have said or have been interpreted as having said, it is not necessarily wrong to treat people as a means to one's own ends. It depends on the sort of treatment involved. To treat some features, aspects or services of a person as a means to one's ends is not necessarily to treat the person wrongly, disrespectfully nor inappropriately.

If we pay our dentist for the desired dental treatment, then the situation does not necessarily become 'positively exploitative'. It might be exploitative if, for instance, we refuse to pay for the good dental treatment which we obtained or if the dentist over-charges or gives bad treatment. However, the situation is not inherently nor essentially exploitative. What is said here about the services provided by a commercial dentist might be said about the services provided by a commercial surrogate mother. That the woman is paid for the services she provides does not imply – nor, to our minds, even suggest – that she is being treated wrongly as a person and/nor merely as a means to someone else's ends. The services which she provides are, from her perspective, the means to ends of her own.

The Brazier Report

The Brazier Report (1998) recommended that surrogate mothers should be paid by commissioning parents only in regard to actual expenses caused by the pregnancy and that section 1A of the 1985 Surrogacy Act which states that surrogate motherhood contracts are not legally enforceable should continue. Also, it recommended that only 'nonprofits making' surrogate motherhood agencies should be legally allowed.

Among the reasons which Brazier *et al.* put forward in support of these recommendations is that C.S.M. is or is likely to become exploitative[3]. Here again, it is not clear what Brazier *et al.* mean by 'exploitation'. Neither is it clear whether the risky transactions they mention as being exploitative can be considered as exploitative. However, whether they are or not exploitative, Brazier *et al.* do not demonstrate that they should be illegal.

Brazier *et al.* sometimes use the term 'exploitation' in what seems like a usual way as, for instance, when they state that 'Payment for their services does not make people into mere means: on the contrary lack of payment (as is slavery or breadline wages) may be much more exploitative' (1998, p.35). More typically, however, they relate the notion of 'exploitation' to that of 'risk' in a way which is very obscure. Pivotal to their case for making C.S.M. illegal are the following passages:

'Even where there is a risk in an occupation (e.g. working as a soldier, or in the police or fire service) payment does not in itself necessarily constitute exploitation. There is unlikely to be exploitation providing that people choosing to undertake such jobs do so with their full knowledge and understanding of such risks, and that the payments made to them are not of a nature or at a level to induce them to take such risks against their better judgement' (1998, p.35).

This seems to imply the very curious suggestion that if, for example, a famous footballer named David Beckham is offered millions of pounds to take the unknown and unknowable risk of crippling himself by playing football for a very good team, then he is more likely thereby to be exploited than is some less talented person who risks injury by playing football for a less well known team for far less money.

Imagine a football player, C, who was as good as Beckham but differed from him in not having a rich wife. It would be more 'exploitative' (or more likely to be 'exploitative') were the very good team to employ C rather than Beckham to play for them since C, more than Beckham, needs the money. This would seem to be another bizarre implication of the view of Brazier *et al.*

The Report continues:

'The issue of exploitation of the surrogate [mother] therefore resolves into the fundamental question of her capacity to foresee the risks entailed. Payment increases the risk of exploitation if it constitutes an inducement to participate in an activity whose degree of risk the surrogate [mother] cannot, in the nature of things, fully understand or predict.' (1998, p.35).

But the questions: Is something or other exploitative? Does it produce a risk of exploitation? Whether exploitative or not, is it risky? are related to separate matters which, in the Brazier Report, tend to be conflated. For instance, marriage can be exploitative since to marry might be to risk exploitation. This does not mean that marriage is inherently exploitative (nor, of course, that it should be illegal). Indeed, life is also potentially risky and exploitative.

If what Brazier *et al.* suggest is correct then it would be arguable that all paid employment is exploitative since, in general, people cannot predict with any certainty that, for example, their place of work will not go on fire nor that they will not be injured on their way to their employment. However, what they suggest does not seem to be correct. At least, in normal usages of the term and in specialist usages of which we are aware, 'exploitation' does not essentially pertain to the failure to be aware of, nor the failure to foresee, hazards or risks.

It is wrong (whether or not it is 'exploitation' and whether or not it should be, illegal) unfairly and/or unjustly to expose people to risks and to misrepresent to them the true nature of risky transactions into which they might enter with us. However, it is not in itself wrong (nor unjust nor unfair) to transact with someone who voluntarily runs a risk with the transaction. Furthermore, such transactions should not necessarily be illegal.

For example, consider the situation of buying and selling houses. Risk and uncertainty are part and parcel of such transactions. Such transactions are sometimes fraudulent and exploitative but they are not always so and the risk and uncertainty do not make them inherently so. If one buys a house, one often runs the risk that the neighbourhood and/or neighbours (and sometimes, even the very house) will subsequently and unpredictably change in such a way that what promised to be an attractive home becomes a problematic one. Such is life but such is not exploitation. Even if one comes to be exploited by one's new neighbours, one was not necessarily exploited by the person who sold the house or by the transaction which constituted the sale. People are, we would agree, exploited if they are persuaded to take a risk which they would not otherwise take on the basis of deliberately misleading information given to them by the party with whom they transact. The party acts unjustly and/or unfairly in this instance. However, if people are persuaded to take a risk which they would not otherwise take by the offer of money, we do not see why this should be said to be exploitative. The other party here is not necessarily acting unjustly nor unfairly by offering the money.

There are, we think, some risks that people should not encourage or allow other people to take. There are also, we think, some risks that people should not legally be allowed to encourage other people to take. However, we do not believe that C.S.M. comes into either category.

Imagine that a person or consortium of people paid some individuals to play Russian roulette for the bizarre pleasure of watching them do it. We would regard this commercial Russian roulette playing as wrong and condemn the commissioning parties for encouraging it. But though we think that this would be wrong it is not exploitative provided that the participants were known to be normal adult human beings who understood, in the normal way, the nature of the risks of the game.

A footballer who is not fully fit might, for the sake of glory and the bonus cup-money, risk permanent injury to himself by playing when it would be wiser to rest. We would not consider this to be exploitation. Thus, to be offered an attractive incentive to do something and, voluntarily and unwisely, to succumb to it is not the same as doing something which someone else wants us to do because he unfairly and/or unjustly pressurises us into doing it. If the unfit player plays because his trainer lies to him about his fitness to play or threatens to molest him unless he plays, that would be another matter.

Notice that a footballer might, for the sake of glory and money, have a career as a professional player and suffer permanent injury or even death on the field or even on the way to or from the field. This would not demonstrate that the decision to become a professional footballer was an unwise one rather than an unlucky one. It certainly would not establish that professional football should be made illegal. Also, notice that to say that payment for particular actions can make people overlook the risks of the actions is only to give part of the picture. Payment can also alter the rationality and wisdom of accepting the risks involved. Consider again commercial Russian roulette. Is there perhaps a price for all or most of us – £100 billion ? – at or above which one would act irrationally and unwisely were one not to play ?

To return to the Brazier Report, it was suggested that:

'We are concerned, however, that women may be entering into surrogacy arrangements without full awareness of the physical and psychological risks... There is evidence that the majority of surrogate [mothers] are significantly poorer than commissioning couples and have relatively low educational attainments.' (p.34).

This suggested poorer status does not have the relevance that Brazier *et al.* claim it has, even in terms of their own argument. If the footballer David Beckham is exploited by receiving money to play football, whether he receives money from people who are richer or poorer than himself is beside the point. Similarly, if the inducement of money rendered commercial surrogate motherhood exploitative, why would it matter where the money came from? For instance, in terms of the argument of Brazier *et al.*, if the money was paid by the state rather than by the commissioning parents, the commercial surrogate mothers would be equally 'exploited' in both cases since they would be equally induced by money to do something which is risky and/or uncertain and something which they would not have done were it not for the money.

If, as Brazier *et al.* suggest, women who have little education are not sufficiently clever or knowledgeable enough to decide for themselves whether or not it is wise for them to be commercial surrogate mothers – and this is not a suggestion which we would make nor one we believe – then there might possibly be a case for not allowing women of little education to become commercial surrogate mothers. However; there is no basis here for making commercial surrogate motherhood in general illegal.

People should be aware of the risks they are running when they do various things such as, for instance, play professional football or become commercial surrogate mothers or professional university lecturers. They should not let the thought of the money involved make them overlook such risks. If they do allow themselves to be so blinded then they are unwise: however, they are not thereby exploited. They might be, in their lack of wisdom, vulnerable to exploitation but that is another matter. To act against one's best interest is not the same thing as being exploited and such acts are not invariably caused by exploitation.

Commercial surrogate mothers can know as well as can Brazier *et al.* what the risks and uncertainties of pregnancy and of C.S.M. are. Indeed, they are more aware than Brazier *et al.* whether the risks involved are worth taking even though, like all mothers, they cannot know for certain what the outcomes of their pregnancies will be nor how they will react to them. But commercial surrogate mothers can know enough and with sufficient assurance for a rational, autonomous, adult and (well-enough) informed choice to be made. If complete, absolute and certain knowledge were required for such choices, no one on the planet earth would ever make them. After all, one might say that life itself is a series of activities, experiences and emotions that one '...cannot, in the nature of things, fully understand or predict'.

Conclusion

Sometimes employers may exploit their employees but such exploitation is not inevitable nor inherent in the situation. Employees, similarly, sometimes exploit their employers. However, such possible exploitation is not an argument – not even a weak one – for making employment illegal. In the same way, it may happen that commissioning parents and/or C.S.M. agencies exploit surrogate mothers. It may even happen that surrogate mothers exploit commissioning parents and/or C.S.M. agencies. But this is not good enough an argument for making C.S.M. illegal [4].

Thus, not all actions which are potentially exploitative and not all exploitations as such should be made illegal. As Wertheimer says:

'Just because an activity is damaging to those who participate in it, it certainly does not follow that the state is justified in prohibiting that activity. We need not be rigorous antipaternalists to believe that there is at least a strong presumption against state interference with consensual activities' (1996, p.306).

Furthermore, the arguments which we have looked at here do not establish that C.S.M. is in principle exploitative or that in practice it is particularly likely to be exploitative. The case against it that we examined, which purports to be about 'exploitation', is not about protecting people from ill-usage by other people but about forcing them to act contrary to their inclinations and in line with the inclinations of those who propose it. This is particularly the case when considering the Brazier report.

Paternalistic intervention might be justified when it is akin, for instance, to stopping people walking over a cliff where the danger, seen by the paternalists, is not apparent to the walkers. However, the arguments we have looked at here concerning C.S.M. are not of the same kind. It is more akin to walkers wanting to walk a different path from the path which the interveners want them to walk and where the dangers are no better known by the interveners than by the walkers

*By Hugh V. McLachlan and J. Kim Swales from *Human Reproduction and Genetic Ethics*, Vol. 7, No. 1, 2001, pp. 8-14.

Footnotes

(1) We discuss some of Anderson's other arguments against C.S.M. in McLachlan and Swales, 2000a. See also McLachlan, 1997.

(2) Note that we disagree strongly with the view that C.S.M. is the buying and selling of children rather than the services of the carrying mother and, sometimes, also those of C.S.M. agencies. See McLachlan and Swales 2000a and McLachlan and Swales, 2000b.

(3) See McLachlan and Swales, 2000a, where other objections to C.S.M. raised by Brazier *et al.* are discussed. See also McLachlan and Swales, 2000b.

(4) Illegal C.S.M. arrangements and contracts which are not legally enforceable are an obvious source of possible exploitation. If one is concerned about exploitation in relation to C.S.M. then perhaps one should be arguing for its legalisation and for reasonable and fair commercial surrogate contracts and agreements that are reasonably and fairly upheld by the courts (see McLachlan and Swales, 2000a).

References

Anderson, Elizabeth, 1993, *Value in Ethics and Economics,* Harvard University Press/The MIT Press.

Brazier, Margaret, *et al.* 1998, *Surrogacy : Review for Health Ministers of Current Arrangements for Payments and Regulations ; Report of the Review Team.* Cm 4068.

Hindess, Barry, 1982, 'Power, Interests and the Outcome of Struggles', *Sociology,* Vol. 16, No. 4

Levine, David P., 1997, *Self-Seeking and the Pursuit of Justice.* Ashgate, Aldershot.

McLachlan, Hugh V., 1997, 'Defending commercial Surrogate Motherhood Against Van Niekerk and Van Zyl, *Journal of Medical Ethics.* Vol. 23, No. 6.

McLachlan, Hugh V., 1998, 'Justice, Rights and Health care: A Discussion of the Report of the Commission on Social Justice' *International Journal of Sociology and Social Policy,* Vol. 9, No. 2.

McLachlan, Hugh V. and Swales, J.K., 2000a, 'Babies, Child Bearers and Commodification : Anderson, Brazier *et al.* and the Political Economy of Commercial Surrogate Motherhood', *Health Care Analysis.* Vol. 8, No. 1.

McLachlan, Hugh V. and Swales, J.K., 2000b, 'Scotland, the Church and Surrogate Motherhood', *Scottish Affairs*. No. 32, Summer.
Scruton, Roger, 1982, *A Dictionary of Political Thought*. Pan Books.
Tong, Rosemary, 1997, *Feminist Approaches to Bioethics*. Westview Press, Oxford.
Warnock, Mary, 1985, *A Question of Life : The Warnock Report on Human Fertilisation and Embryology*. Basil Blackwell, Oxford.
Wertheimer, Alan, 1996, *Exploitation.* Princeton University Press, Princeton.

Chapter Thirteen

Surrogate Motherhood, Rights and Duties: A Reply to Campbell*

Abstract.

In a recent article in Health Care Analysis (Vol. 8, No. 1), Campbell misrepresents our specific arguments about commercial surrogate motherhood (C.S.M.) and our general philosophical and political views by saying or suggesting that we are 'Millsian' liberals and consequentialists. He gives too the false impression that we do not oppose, in principle, slavery and child purchase. Here our position on C.S.M. is re-expressed and elaborated upon in order to eliminate possible confusion. Our general ethical and philosophical framework is also outlined and shown to be other than Campbell says that it is. In particular, a moral philosophy that is based on neither consequentialism nor Kantianism is presented. C.S.M., it is argued, is not child purchase. It is like it in some respects and unlike it in others. It is unlike it in the respects which, relative to the present discussion, matter.

Key words: *child purchase, commercial surrogate motherhood, commodification, consequentialism, Kantianism*

Campbell (2000) misrepresents our specific arguments about commercial surrogate motherhood (C.S.M.) and our general philosophical and political views by saying or suggesting that we are 'Millsian' liberals and consequentialists.[1] He gives too the false impression that we do not oppose, in principle, slavery and child purchase.

Our position, as presented in the article under discussion might be expressed, or re-expressed, as follows. The arguments of Anderson and of Brazier *et al.* in relation to 'commodification' do not establish that C.S.M. is, because of its consequences, wrong. We do not think that, on grounds other than consequences, C.S.M. is wrong but it might be. The arguments of Anderson and of Brazier *et al.* in relation to 'commodification' do not show that C.S.M. is a breach of a mother's maternal duty but other arguments might show that C.S.M. is in breach of that or of some moral principle.

We do not think that it is merely the consequences of actions which render them right or wrong. For instance, an act of adultery, even if it had good consequences, might be wrong because it breaches the principle that you ought not to do what you promised not to do.

However, it does not follow that adultery should be a crime. Similarly even if, because of its consequences or on some other grounds, C.S.M. is morally wrong, it does not follow that it should be a crime. Even if it would be *legitimate* for the state to have laws against adultery and C.S.M. – and, as non-Millians, we are not addressing that particular issue – it would not, in our view, be wise, at least in the context of Britain, to have them.

Campbell writes: '... I am willing to be convinced that, after all, there is no real risk in a free market in parenthood' (2000, pp. 39-40). We hope that he is not brought to this view by anything that we wrote. We are not in favour of the buying and selling *of parenthood* (and nor of the buying and selling of *children)*. We do not advocate a market – whether or not a 'free' one – in parenthood (nor in children). We are not against the buying and selling of the services of a carrying mother and it is the exchange of money *for this service* wherein, in our view, the essence of commercial surrogate motherhood lies. One of the advantages of making C.S.M. contracts legal would be the specification of exactly what is being bought and sold. Whether refraining from pursuing the claim to legal rights of parenthood, which is not the same as reneging on the moral duties that one has concerning it, should be (as we suggested) legally buyable and sellable is debatable. It is, in any case, not pivotal to the issue of C.S.M.

Campbell writes:

'In our era, the combination of a Millsian liberalism and a postmodern scepticism about communal norms makes the kinds of arguments espoused by McLachlan and Swales ... sound much more reasonable and persuasive than such claims to the priority of parental duty over freedom to trade ... Defenders of the liberal view of autonomy shift the burden of proof the other way. In the style of John Stuart Mill, they demand clear evidence of harm (to child or surrogate mother) before we are entitled to interfere in the liberty of commissioning couples and surrogate mothers to trade parental options.' (Campbell, 2000, p. 36)

This is not our view. What we said was that the onus is on those who propose making and/or keeping C.S.M. illegal to justifying the legal restriction rather than on those who are against that particular legal restriction to justify its absence. There might well be a justification for the legislation. What Anderson and Brazier *et al.* say about 'commodification' does not, in our view, constitute one: that was the essence of our piece. (Other issues, notably that of alleged 'exploitation', arise in the debate about C.S.M. See, for instance, McLachlan and Swales, 2000b.)

We did not say that the only possible justification of the legislation is a Millian nor do we believe it to be. It might well turn our that a non-Millian justification for the illegality of C.S.M. will be put forward. We see no reason for rejecting the possibility *a priori*. For instance, if we reject aspects of the case of, say, Brazier *et al.* as a weak paternalistic argument, it does not follow that we are, like Mill, against paternalism as such; perhaps a stronger paternalistic argument against C.S.M. would, were one to be presentable, convince us.[2]

It is specifically not our view that it is harm merely to the child or to the surrogate mother which could justify the illegality of C.S.M. We wrote:

'It could turn out that there are good reasons for making C.S.M. illegal. Brazier *et al.* talk as if the only relevant interests concerned here were those of the parties directly concerned ... We think that the proper target of public policy lies elsewhere. For instance, if it could be shown that children born by commercial surrogate mothers are particularly delinquent and, throughout their lives, a burden to the other members of their societies, then there might well be at least the basis of a powerful case for illegalising C.S.M.' (McLachlan and Swales, 2000a, p. 16)

It is inaccurate to call us Millian liberals. It is inaccurate and, to us, offensive to suggest that we are consequentialists. Campbell writes:

'... brides cannot be purchased, nor can children; and although the rights and duties of parenthood can be voluntarily relinquished, they cannot be sold or purchased. These institutional arrangements are based on an understanding of the moral character of the relationships themselves, and are not dependent simply on a prediction of good and bad consequences. They are grounded in non-consequential arguments of a similar kind to those which oppose slavery in principle. For those who believe that only consequentialist arguments are truly rational and convincing, such assumptions will be questioned by use of the "happy slave" type of counter argument.' (Campbell, 2000, p. 37)

There are, or might be, consequentialist grounds for and against thinking that C.S.M. is immoral just as there are or might be non-consequentialist grounds for thinking the same things. Campbell is relying upon a false dichotomy here. The 'moral principles' which he alludes to do not all or necessarily point in the one direction. Even if Campbell is right in saying that there is a moral principle relating to parental duty which tends to push C.S.M. out of moral bounds, the principle of favouring and fostering human autonomy, (and not merely that one) pulls in the other direction.[3]

Similarly, one might accept some consequentialist arguments without being a consequentialist i.e. without believing that only consequentialist arguments should count. Campbell might be thought to deny this when he says:

... consequentialist arguments are rational and convincing only to those who accept their assumptions. To others, their treasure chest of the components of human goodness seems sadly empty. (Campbell, 2000, p. 37)

One is not compelled to choose between consequentialism and non-consequentialism. That by virtue of which good actions are good actions is not necessarily the same in all instances. Some good actions are good because of their consequences. Some good actions are good ones for other reasons. Utilitarianism gives a correct account of the ethics of some actions. Kantianism gives a correct account of the ethics of others. Some actions are not correctly accounted for by either utilitarianism or Kantianism. Some are accounted for correctly by a combination of both. So, at least, is what we think.[4] We might be wrong in thinking this but we would rather be known for thinking it than be wrongly thought of as thinking something else and, in particular, as being consequentialists.

A distinction too should be made between consequentialism in relation to ethics and consequentialism in relation to public policies. One might think that public policies are to be justified or condemned solely in terms of their consequences without thinking that actions are morally good or morally bad ones solely because of their consequences.

In relation to ethics in particular, we are definitely not consequentialists. For instance, we wrote in an article unrelated to C.S.M. that: 'Often, it matters not merely what is done but why it is done' (McLachlan and Swales, 1999, p. 7). We wrote too that:

'... it is not a ludicrous point of view that there are some sorts of decisions that people ought not to make no matter what are the consequences of failure to make them. Sometimes, when people perform their duties and do, in particular circumstances what they ought to do – and this might be to refuse to make a particular sort of decision – the outcome can seem to be ludicrous. Yet, to do their duty in such circumstances is, perhaps, what people ought to do.' (McLachlan and Swales, 1999, p. 7)

This hardly sounds like consequentialism.

We are 'alldependsists'.[5] We are not sceptics, relativists or postmodernists. We think that the short, correct answer to all or, at least, to most philosophical questions is: it all depends. When an action is a good one or a bad one, by virtue of which is it such? It all depends. When one knows that X is true, how does one know? It all depends. What is it to be an X, when an X is a class term such as 'table', 'horse' or 'game'? It all depends. Essentialism gives a correct account of some universal terms. Nominalism gives a correct account of some others. Yet more are correctly accounted for by neither of these theories. When, to quote Mill, are '... mankind warranted, individually or collectively, in interfering with the liberty of action of any of their number ...'? (Mill, 1966, p. 135). Mill says that the question can be given a general answer in terms of 'one very simple principle', namely: 'self protection'. We say: it all depends.

Campbell paints us as consequentialists and as not being against child purchase in principle when he says the following:

'... they ... go on to state that: "Even if it were the purchase of a child, as long as the child were treated subsequently as a child should be treated, the 'commodification' involved might be excusable, or, even, laudable" (p. 23) Thus it appears from this statement that they see no objection in principle to child purchase, provided good consequences come of it.' (Campbell, 2000, p. 36)

This is not what we say and we are surprised to be told that it appears from what we say. To talk of a child being treated as a child should be treated is not to talk merely about the *effects* of the treatment of the child.

There are objections in principle to child purchase. Actions are often simultaneously in accord with and in conflict with a variety of principles. There are objections in principle, say, to telling lies and killing people yet even when they involve telling lies and killing people some actions – think, say, of the Second World War and some of the events which comprised it -are excusable and, even laudable.

There might well be objections on the basis of various principles – for instance, the principle that the state should not encourage or appear to encourage sex outside marriage and the principle that those who use something, rather than those who do not, should pay for it – to the distribution by the state of free condoms even if in some circumstances – such, say, as exist in South Africa at present in relation to Aids – the distribution might, because of its possible consequences, be justifiable.

We stress the qualification *even if it were the purchase of a child.* C.S.M. is not, for reasons which we outline in our article, the purchase of a child. As a matter of legal fact, in, for instance, Britain, the purchase of a child is an impossibility. And so it should be.

The point is that we see – because, in our view, Anderson and Brazier *et al.* have shown none – no objection in any principle pertaining to commodification to commercial surrogate motherhood. C.S.M. is not child purchase. If it were, there would be an objection in principle to it. Even then, on the basis of other principles and/or the consequences of it C.S.M. might still be justifiable either in general or in particular instances.

According to Campbell:

'We – with the possible exception of McLachlan and Swales – already accept that child purchase and financial rewards for giving up one's child for adoption are morally wrong and must be illegal.' (Campbell, 2000, p. 37)

Child purchase is morally wrong and also must be illegal. We oppose child purchase just as we oppose slavery in principle (and in other relevant ways as well). What might be and seems to be at issue between Campbell and us is the nature of the principle or principles concerned. Slavery as slavery is, as we said, wrong: we suggested that it was not the issue of money changing hands that constitutes the wrongness of slavery. Similarly, we suggested that the exchange of money does not render C.S.M. wrong. It certainly does not make it slavery. It does not constitute child purchase in the way that an exchange of money in particular circumstances can constitute, say, house purchase.

C.S.M. is, in some respects, like wrong things. However, it is unlike them in other respects and not like them in the respects which, morally, matter. There is a story told of shipwrecked sailors who were on a life-raft. They realised that the life-raft too was sinking. Death seemed imminent. 'Do something religious', one of them said: 'Do something religious'. In response, another of the doomed men took a collection. The association of ideas is, as Hume indicated long ago, a powerful psychological phenomenon. However, the collecting of donated money will not in itself render an action an appropriate and a good one any more than the commercial exchange of money will render it an inappropriate and a bad one.

*By Hugh V. McLachlan and J. Kim Swales, from *Health Care Analysis,* 2001, Vol. 9, No. 1, pp. 101-107. With kind permission of Springer Sciences and Business Media.

Notes

(1) See Campbell, 2000 and McLachlan and Swales, 2000a.
(2) See McLachlan and Swales, 2000b.
(3) See McLachlan, 1997.
(4) See McLachlan, 1981.
(5) See McLachlan and Swales, 1998.

References

Campbell, A.V., (2000) Surrogacy, Rights and Duties: A Partial Commentary. *Health Care Analysis* 8, 35-40.

McLachlan, H.V. (1981) Wittgenstein, Family Resemblances and the Theory of Classification. *International Journal of Sociology and Social Policy* 1(1), 1-16.

McLachlan, H.V. (1997) Defending Commercial Surrogate Motherhood Against Van Nierkerk and Van Zyl. *Journal of Medical Ethics* 23, 344-348.

McLachlan, H.V. and Swales, J.K. (1998) The Methodology Rather than the Rhetoric of Economics: McCloskey on Popper and Hume. *Journal of Interdisciplinary Economics* 9(2), 125-143.

McLachlan, H.V. and Swales, J.K. (1999) A Drunk Driver, A Sober Pedestrian and the Allocation of Tragically Scarce and Indivisible Emergency Hospital Treatment. *Health Care Analysis 7(1), 5-21.*

McLachlan, H.V. and Swales, J.K. (2000a) Babies, Child Bearers and Commodification: Anderson, Brazier *et al.* and the Political Economy of Commercial Surrogate Motherhood. *Health Care Analysis* 8(1), 1-18.

McLachlan, H.V. and Swales, J.K. (2000b) Scotland, the Church and Surrogate Motherhood. *Scottish Affairs* (Summer) (32).

Mill, J.S. (1966) On Liberty. In M. Warnock (Ed.), *Utilitarianism.* London: Collins.

Chapter Fourteen

Surrogate Motherhood: Beyond the Warnock and the Brazier Reports*

Introduction

The law in Britain regarding surrogate motherhood requires to be reconsidered and more deeply pondered on than it has been hitherto. In saying this, we are strongly of the view that in the framing and implementation of public policy, of crucial importance is not only what is done but also why what is done is done. We shall look at the deliberations concerning surrogate motherhood of the Warnock Report on Human Fertilisation and Embryology (1984) and at the Brazier Report on Surrogacy (1998). The debate within these documents is – in both cases – unsatisfactory, insufficiently comprehensive and lacking in rigour and balance. The argumentation that is presented in these reports does not resolve the issues: neither the present legal position nor a suggested alternative one is sustained by it.

Britain was the first country in the world to have legislation specifically about surrogate motherhood when, as what seemed like a panic measure, in 1985, The Surrogacy Arrangements Act was passed. Under this Act, although it is not a crime to be a surrogate mother or to be a commissioning parent (whether or not money changes hands in the arrangement) 'commercial' surrogate agencies and the 'commercial' actions of surrogacy agents were prohibited. It was stated in section 36(1) of the Human Fertilisation and Embryology Act of 1990 that no surrogate motherhood arrangement is enforceable by or against any of the people making it. In 1995, section 30 of the same Act came into force. The effect of this is that married couples who have commissioned a 'surrogate mother' to carry a child for them may apply for and be granted a parental order. By virtue of this they will be regarded as the legal parents of the child provided that one or both of them supplied the gametes of the embryo of the child. A further stipulation is that the court must be satisfied that no money or equivalent benefit, other than 'for expenses reasonably incurred' has been given or received by the husband or wife pertaining to the arrangement unless authorised by the court.

The impetus for this legislation – although the legislation and Warnock's recommendations diverged to an extent – came from the Warnock Report on Human Fertilisation and Embryology (1984, reprinted in Warnock, 1985). Therein, surrogate motherhood is discussed very briefly, almost in passing. The treatment of the issue consists of six pages (plus an expression of dissent of two and a half pages) out of the eighty nine pages of the Report. Their recommendations and the *rationale* for them are, we shall show, unsatisfactory.

According to McHale *et al.*(1999, pp. 636-637):

'Commentators are virtually unanimous that the Warnock Committee's recommendations on surrogacy represent the weakest stage of the report, since the conclusions appear to have been based on public opposition to the practice rather than any considered philosophical position'.

Further, as Freeman notes, Warnock's recommendation concerning surrogate motherhood are very paternalistic and this paternalism is at variance with the tone of the other recommendations of the Warnock Report in relation, say, to I.V.F. and embryo donation, where the virtues of autonomy and self-determination are upheld. (See Freeman, 1989 and McLachlan, 1993)

The Warnock Report

Concerning surrogate motherhood, the Warnock Committee made two majority recommendations. One was that all surrogate motherhood agreements – not only commercial ones -should be illegal contracts and therefore unenforceable in the courts. They made this recommendation – to put the matter 'beyond any possible doubt in law' – even although they felt that surrogate motherhood arrangement were probably not enforceable anyway. The other was that the creation and operation of agencies (both 'profit making' and non – 'profit making' ones) "... whose purposes include the recruitment of women for surrogate pregnancy or making arrangements for individuals or couples who wish to utilise the services of a carrying mother should be a criminal offence. (See Warnock, 1985, p. 47)

As we have seen, the present law in the U.K. is in accord with the first but not with the second recommendation.

The *rationale* given by Warnock (1985, p. 46) for these recommendations is weak. It is as follows:

'That people should treat others as a means to their own ends, however desirable the consequences, must always be liable to moral objection. Such treatment of one person by another becomes positively exploitative when financial interests are involved. It is therefore with the commercial exploitation of surrogacy that we have been primarily, but by no means exclusively concerned.'

There is an allusion to Kant here. According to Kant – and Kant was not infallible! – it is morally wrong to treat people merely as means to one's own ends. However, not even Kant would say that it is always wrong to treat people as means to our own ends: such actions can be right as long as they are consistent with treating the people concerned with the respect due to autonomous moral agents. Surrogate motherhood can fulfil this condition. Furthermore, it can hardly have been Kant's view that all morally wrong actions should be made crimes. Kant thought that, for instance, suicide is a highly immoral action. Even if Kant were right so to think, would it be wise to make suicide – as it was before – a crime?

One treats a dentist as a means to one's own ends when one pays a dentist for the very intimate services of dental treatment. Unless the dentist is coerced by the patient or the patient's friends into performing the service or isn't paid for it, there seems to be no reason for imagining that such a commercial transaction is exploitative or in any way morally dubious. If contractual agreements between patients and dentist were legally unenforceable and/or if commercial dental agencies were illegal then one can readily see that visits to dental surgeries might be more hazardous and worrying than they presently are.

Warnock does not make it at all clear what is meant by 'exploitation' or why she thinks that surrogate motherhood, especially 'commercial' surrogate motherhood is exploitative. (See Wertheimer, 1996 and McLachlan and Swales, 2000a and 2001b) Furthermore, even if commercial surrogate motherhood were exploitative, a case would still have to be made for saying that it should be illegal. Consider, for instance, Marxists. They think that members of the proletariat are being exploited when they work for the bourgeoisie. However, they do not argue that it should be a crime for the bourgeoisie to employ people or to advertise their services as employers as so forth. Nor do they say that commercial employment contracts should be legally unenforceable. Perhaps the world would be a better place were there no capitalist employers and no surrogate mothers (and perhaps it would not be). But public policies have to be made for how conditions are now, rather than for how they might be or would, if the best came to the best, be.

In the U.K., exploitation is not in itself a criminal offence. To our knowledge, exploitation is nowhere a criminal offence. If Warnock thinks that commercial surrogate motherhood should be criminal because it is exploitative, why does she not argue that exploitation should be a crime? If it is not appropriate to make exploitation a crime, then it is not at all clear why it should be appropriate to make commercial surrogate motherhood a crime on the grounds of its supposed exploitativeness.

In a sketchy, hit-or-miss sort of a way, the Warnock Report very briefly outlines, with no critical evaluation at all, some 'arguments against surrogacy' and some 'arguments for surrogacy'. This exercise is beside the point. One might as well put arguments for and against, say, the consumption of alcohol or the committing of adultery. Should such activities be illegal? That is another matter. Whether it is wise to be or to use the services of a surrogate mother is not what is at issue. One need not put forward a convincing case for adultery or for alcohol consumption in order to justify the legality of the practices. They should be legal unless and until a good case can be given for making them illegal. Similarly, surrogate motherhood, including commercial surrogate motherhood should be legal unless a case can be established for making it illegal. There is no onus on those who think it should not be illegal to establish a case for not outlawing it.

'The moral and social objections to surrogacy have weighed heavily with us': so it is said in the Warnock Report. (Warnock, 1985, p.46) What is not clear is why the suggested moral objections weighed so heavily. In seeming to give, as it were, the pros and cons of surrogate motherhood, it might seem that the Warnock Report is even-handed in its treatment on the topic. In our view this is not so. For instance, it is said that:

'There are strongly held objections to the concept of surrogacy, and it seems from the evidence submitted to us that the weight of public opinion is against the practice. The objections turn essentially on the view that to introduce a third party into the process of procreation which should be confined to the loving partnership between two people, is an attack on the value of the marital relationship'. (Warnock, 1985. p. 44)

How could this objection, even if one accepted it, support the contention that surrogate motherhood agreements should be illegal, legally unenforceable contracts and that commercial surrogate motherhood agencies should be illegal? In any case, not everyone accepts this view of the marital relationship as the solely appropriate one for the procreation and rearing of children. Warnock was, in the early 1980s, probably wrong in her estimates as to what public opinion regarding surrogate motherhood and regarding marriage was. Public opinion has changed since then and not in the direction of affording marriage a uniquely favoured position concerning the procreation and rearing of children. (See Brazier *et al.*, 1998)

Furthermore, to regard surrogate motherhood as an 'attack' on marriage is bizarre. 'Surrogate' is a synonym for 'substitute' and, by convention the word 'surrogate' rather than the more usual word, 'substitute', is used in this context. The terminology requires clarification. There are two sorts of so-called 'surrogate motherhood': genetic and gestational. In the former one, the male member of the commissioning couple impregnates – usually via artificial insemination – the surrogate mother who is the genetic mother of the child. In the latter one, the male member of the couple fertilises, *in vitro,* an egg from the female member of the couple. The fertilised egg is placed, for development and delivery, into the womb of the surrogate mother, who is not genetically related to the child at all. She is not a substitute for a mother, she is someone who performs for the mother the service – which function the mother cannot perform for herself – of carrying her baby (i.e. the baby of the genetic mother) to term. The service is a substitute for the function: one woman is not a substitute for the other. In the former case – that of genetic surrogate motherhood – the so-called surrogate mother is the mother of the child (both biologically and legally) and the female of the commissioning couple is the one who, strictly speaking, becomes the surrogate – i.e. substitute – mother. While she is not and never can become the biological mother of the child, she can become its legal mother and be, as is said, its social mother.

Suppose that a husband and wife want to have a child of their own but that the woman, although fertile, has a damaged womb. Suppose that they decide that they want to use the services of a gestational, carrying, so-called 'surrogate-mother'. Suppose too that they are happy to pay money to a surrogate motherhood agency in order to make and keep contact with someone who they consider appropriate for the performance of the particular service. Perhaps they have no friends or relatives to whom they would want to be indebted for the performance of such a service for them, although they might have an abundance of relatives and friends.

In these circumstances, there is no obvious reason why one should say that 'surrogate-motherhood' is an attack on the marriage in this illustrative example (nor an attack on any one else's marriage). If anything, it seems supportive of, rather than antagonistic to, the relationship of the commissioning couple. You might say that, for instance, adultery is an attack on marriages in general or particular. However, this is not akin to adultery. Furthermore, that adultery should be illegal because it is an attack on marriage is not a view that is sufficiently widely held in contemporary Britain to require to be seriously addressed, although it is very firmly held by some.

Even with genetic surrogate motherhood, it is far from clear that it is likely to undermine marriage in general or in particular. Given the prevalent high divorce rate, it is strange even to talk about such a consideration as this. Of course, having a child in these circumstances might drive a couple apart but getting married, with or without children, and having children, with or without marriage, can drive some couples apart: this hardly seem like an argument against the legality of marriage nor the legality of having children.

The Warnock Report itself also says: 'As for intrusion into the marriage relationship, it is argued that those who feel strongly about this need not seek such treatment, but they should not seek to prevent others from having access to it'. (Warnock, 1985, p. 46) This seems to us to be a sound point and one which itself answers the suggested fulcrum of objections to surrogate motherhood.

The arguments for and against legislation concerning surrogate motherhood are not, in the Warnock Report, rigorously, rationally, impartially and judiciously weighed. For instance, as an objection to surrogate motherhood it is said: 'Furthermore, it is felt that a surrogacy agreement is degrading to the child who is to be the outcome of it since, for all practical purpose, the child will have been bought for money'. (Warnock, 1985, p. 45) This is all that is said about this point: there is no attempt to develop it or to evaluate it critically. The point, as it stands, is a facile one. Is it better not to be born at all than to be degraded? Should it be illegal to degrade people? Is it degrading to be the outcome of a commercial surrogate motherhood agreement? 'For all practical purposes', the child will have been born when otherwise it would not have been. Is not that the crucial point? Furthermore, as we shall argue more fully later, commercial surrogate motherhood is not the purchase of children: it is, if it is the actual purchase of anything at all, the purchase of something other than that such as, say, the services of the carrying mother. To say that 'for all practical purposes', this is the purchase of children is like saying that rape is, for all practical purposes, the same as seduction or that stealing is, for all practical purposes, the same as receiving something as a gift. Often, even when outcomes are, in some respects, similar, what matters hugely is how the similar outcomes have dissimilar means of bringing them about.

The arguments given in the Warnock Report against surrogate motherhood amount, in essence, to the claim that it is felt to be ethically unacceptable. There are various problems with this position. If Warnock and others feel that surrogate motherhood is ethically unacceptable then the solution for them is obvious. They need not indulge in it. Other people feel differently about it. Why should their actions be constrained by the feelings – and, if you like, by the 'values' – of Warnock and others? The reasons given and mentioned by Warnock for supposing that surrogate motherhood is ethically unacceptable are not good ones. Furthermore, to say that something is 'ethically unacceptable' is not to say that it should be illegal. Adultery and the over-enthusiastic consumption of alcohol, for instance, can be ethically unacceptable. It does not follow that it would be wise to make these activities or the actions of professionals and others who facilitate them criminal offences. Why should surrogate motherhood and commercial surrogate motherhood agencies be illegal? Why should surrogate motherhood contracts, including 'commercial' ones, not be legal? These are the questions that are not adequately addressed by the Warnock Report. (See McLachlan, 1997a)

The Warnock Report: Expression of Dissent

There is a minority view also given – by Wendy Greengross and David Davies – as an 'Expression of Dissent[1] from the Warnock Report. The recommendations of the minority are more reasonable or, rather, less unreasonable than the majority ones. However, they are still unjustified in their restrictiveness, whether or not their restrictiveness might, on some grounds or other, be justifiable.

Greengross and Davies are not against the possible legal enforceability of surrogate motherhood agreements. They write:

'If our proposals are accepted, we believe that it would be inappropriate for steps to be taken to provide that all surrogacy agreements are illegal contracts.... For the time being the Courts should be free to consider individual cases on their own merits if they so choose'. (Warnock, 1985, p. 89)

The current law is not in accord with this.

Partially at least, with another of their recommendations, the current law in the U.K. is in accord: 'non-commercial' agencies are not illegal. Greengross and Davies recommended that, under licence (from what has since emerged as the Human Embryology and Fertilisation Authority) and with suitable regulations, surrogate motherhood agencies of some sort, akin to traditional adoption and fostering agencies might be legally allowable. This arrangement was to be allowed provided that: 'there was no commercial motive', although they were prepared to accept that surrogate mothers might be paid for their services. They say: 'On the other hand anyone (including a medical practitioner) who made surrogacy arrangements for a couple and who was not licensed to do so would be committing an offence, regardless of whether they were acting for profit'. (Warnock, 1985, p. 89)

To a large extent, the minority agreed with the majority recommendation concerning 'commercial' surrogate motherhood agencies but disagreed, to an extent, with the majority's *rationale* for it. Greengross and Davies write:

'We go along entirely with our colleagues in our disapproval of surrogacy for convenience. We also agree that the criminal law should be brought in to prevent the operation of profit making agencies in this field, although our reasons for this are somewhat different from those of our colleagues. In our view the question of exploitation of the surrogate mother, or the treating of her as a means to other people's ends, is not as clear cut a moral issue as our colleagues assert.

On the other hand we hold firmly that the very difficult personal, legal and social issues raised by surrogacy lie close to those raised by adoption and fostering and hence there should be no place for commercial operations just as there is no place for commercial adoption agencies.' (Warnock, 1985, p. 87)

This does not actually tell one what their reason is for prohibiting certain types of agencies, only what it is the same as. It would have been interesting if Greengross and Davies had said why they think that 'there is no place for commercial adopting agencies' since their reason might have been a poor one and/or it might have been a reason which did not apply to surrogate motherhood agencies. That it is wise to make the operations of commercial surrogate motherhood agencies illegal has been established by the minority members no more than it has been by the majority members on the Warnock Committee.

The views of the public have not come to a mature decision of the question of surrogate motherhood, said Greengross and Davies. They say too:

'Thus we think it is too early to take a final decision one way or the other. We wish to have the opportunity in the next few years to see what the demand is, whether an agency is prepared to come forward to satisfy it, and whether the consequences are generally acceptable or not. We simply ask that the door be left slightly ajar so that surrogacy can be more effectively assessed'. (Warnock, 1985, p. 89)

How much more sensible than the majority view this is! However, why not go further still? Why leave the door only slightly ajar? Why not allow all sorts of agencies – including, whatever the terms might mean, 'commercial' and 'profit making' ones – to emerge and see what happens? Why not, too, look at the situation in the U.S.A. where, in the various states, different types of surrogate motherhood agencies with different rules and regulations have emerged? Perhaps the 'commercial' agencies will offer better services. (See Galbraith, McLachlan and Swales, 2005)

The Brazier Report

In June 1997, a small team was given the task of reviewing for the U.K. Health Ministers some aspects of the law and its implementation concerning surrogate motherhood. This Review Team comprised: Margaret Brazier, Professor of Law at Manchester University; Alastair Campbell, Professor of Ethics in Medicine at the University of Bristol; and Professor Susan Golombok, Professor of Psychology at the City University, London. It was chaired by Professor Brazier. With remarkable promptness, in October 1998, *Surrogacy: Review For the Health Ministers of Current Arrangements for Payments and Regulations; Report of the Review Team,* Cm 4068 was published.

With good reason, it is said in the Brazier Report: 'We find that the incomplete implementation of the recommendations of either the majority or the minority of the Warnock Committee created a policy vacuum within which surrogacy has developed in a haphazard fashion'. (Brazier *et al.,* 1998, p. i) However, the law and public policy require a more radical re-appraisal than Brazier and her colleagues were authorised to give them. The terms of references of the Review Team were too narrow. They were:

'...to consider whether payments, including expenses, to surrogate mothers should continue to be allowed, and if so on what basis;

to examine whether there is a case for the legislation of surrogacy arrangements through a recognised body or bodies; and if so to advise on the scope and operation of such arrangements;

in the light of the above to advise whether changes are needed to the Surrogacy Arrangements Act 1985 and/or section 30 of the Human Fertilisation and Embryology Act 1990.' (Brazier, *et al.,* 1998, p. 1)

It was specified that it was not the role of the team to consider surrogate motherhood in the round. Tessa Jowell, the Minister for Public Health said:

'We have specifically asked the review team to consider the issue within the context that surrogacy should not be commercialised and that any woman who has a baby as part of a surrogacy arrangement should not be compelled to give it up if she changes her mind. We also want to know whether there is, realistically, any practical way in which surrogacy arrangements could or should be regulated and if so how. (Brazier *et al.*, 1998, p. 1)

Why should the question of whether or not 'commercial' – whatever the term might mean -surrogate motherhood be ruled out of bounds? Why should it not be addressed? It is not as if the matter has already been discussed deeply and for a long period of time and nor is it a manifest, self-evident truth that commercial surrogate motherhood should be illegal. If it is wise that commercial surrogate motherhood is illegal, what is there to fear from an examination of the question? Would not a sound and sensible re-assessment of the illegality of commercial surrogate motherhood show that it should be illegal if it should be illegal?

Similarly, if it is demonstrable that a carrying mother who changes her mind should never be compelled to part with a baby should she change her mind, it would be useful to be reminded of the demonstration. After all, we compel baby sitters and foster parents to surrender children – no matter how attached to them emotionally they might be – to people who are sometimes no more biologically related to the children concerned than they are. In the case of gestational surrogate motherhood, the baby is genetically the child of the commissioning couple: the carrying mother is not genetically related to the child. Even if, normally, carrying mothers should not be legally compelled to surrender their babies – babies of whom it could be said with reference to the commissioning parents that they are 'their' babies – one would want longer to think about the issues. One would want to be made aware of the relevant arguments and considerations before saying with justified confidence that carrying mothers should never be compelled to surrender a carried child. If, too, a woman who has a baby as part of a surrogacy arrangement should not be compelled to give it up if she changes her mind, she should, perhaps, be compelled instead to give up something or other else, even, if only, money. Whether surrogate motherhood should be 'commercialised' and commercial agreements be legal is separable from the question of whether or not a carrying mother should be compelled to give up the baby if she changes her mind. The Minister of Health's attitude here towards disputed babies evokes an image of an ostrich rather than of a Solomon.

Brazier and her colleagues were given a narrow remit. However, they do not inspire confidence in their deliberations when they say:

'Even if our Terms of Reference allowed us to recommend the full commercialisation of surrogacy, we would not do so, because it would imply a normalisation of what we believe to be a difficult personal choice, with an unknown degree of psychological risk.' (Brazier *et al.*, 1998, p. 36)

The Brazier three are willing to make this particular policy recommendation without the benefit of reflection upon the arguments which might have been presented to a review team had they been sought. One is, therefore, led to wonder as to the extent to which the other recommendations they make, in the same breath, are the results of a mature and sympathetic consideration of the arguments that were presented to them.

The Recommendations of the Brazier Report

The Review Team considers that its recommendations are more like the minority than the majority view of the Warnock Report concerning surrogate motherhood. Like the minority, Brazier and her team want to regulate and control surrogate motherhood rather than to ban and/or prevent it completely.

An important part of the background to the setting up of the Review Team headed by Brazier was concern that commissioning couples were – without prior authorisation by the courts – paying carrying mothers more than 'reasonable expenses'. Then, rather than being consequently denied parental orders, commissioning parents were having the payments authorised retrospectively and being granted the orders. The Review Team recommended that this practice should cease. They recommended that parental orders should not be granted to couples who paid more than actual expenses directly relating to the pregnancy and they recommended that what constitutes actual expenses should be defined by a new Surrogacy Act. They recommended that parental orders should be obtainable only in the High Court.

They recommended too that, under the new proposed Act, surrogate motherhood agencies would be legally required to be registered by the Department of Health. They recommend that, as is the case now, only agencies that operate 'on a non-profit making basis' should be legally allowed. To operate a surrogate motherhood agency that was not registered would become a crime. Under the recommendations, as now, it would not be a criminal offence to be a surrogate mother or to use one, whether or not payments above that of expenses changed hands.

It is also their recommendation that a Code of Practice should be produced. This would, in terms of the proposed Surrogacy Act, be legally binding on surrogate motherhood agencies although it would not be binding on the surrogate mothers and commissioning couples. The Team clearly envisages that it would be part of the Code of Practice that commissioning couples do not pay more than (statutorily defined) actual expenses. If they do, then, as we have seen, they should, in terms of the recommendations, be prevented from becoming the legal parents of the carried children concerned. These children – let us not forget – might be the biological children of the over-spending couples. This is obviously a very tough-minded approach. If the proposed legislation were ever passed, it would be most interesting to see how courts would deal with it, given their 'soft' approach to current surrogate motherhood legislation and given what seems to us to be a softening, rather than a hardening, in public opinion towards surrogate motherhood.

Are Brazier's recommendations concerning expenses practicable? Could courts actually operate, even had they a mind to, as Brazier suggests? How could the courts know exactly how much money actually had changed hands if the parties did not want to tell them? Even if the parties did want to tell the courts the truth about how much money changed hands, how could the courts know whether to believe that they were telling the truth even when they were? The courts might be able to establish in some cases – through documentation pertaining to cashed cheques, for instance -that at least such and such an amount was paid by a couple to a woman. But how could they possibly establish in any cases that only such and such an amount changed hands? They could not. Any one who is familiar with the hypocrisy and nonsense about 'amateurism' in sport and athletics -but not only he or she – might well shudder at the thought of courts being dragged into decisions about expenses and the limits of reasonable expenses in relation to surrogate motherhood.

The Review Team recommends for consideration the view that the Surrogacy Arrangements Act 1985 and section 30 of the Human Fertilisation and Embryology Act 1990 should be repealed and replaced with a new act. The proposed Surrogacy Act would include:

'(i) the continuation of the current provisions of Section 1A of the 1985 Act relating to the non-enforceability of the surrogacy contract;

(ii) the continuation of current provisions prohibiting commercial agencies from assisting in the creation of surrogacy arrangements and related provisions prohibiting advertisements in relation to surrogacy arrangements;

(iii) new statutory provisions defining and limiting lawful payments to surrogate mothers;

(iv) provision for the promulgation by the UK Departments of Health of a Code of Practice governing surrogacy arrangements generally;

(v) provision for the registration of non profit-making agencies by the Departments of Health and that such agencies should be required to comply with the Departments' Code of Practice on surrogacy arrangements.

(vi) provision to prohibit the operation of unregistered agencies;

(vii) new provisions for the grant of a parental order to commissioning couples .... The revised order should provide the applicants for a parental order to establish compliance with the Surrogacy Act and the Code of Practice; and that they have complied with the statutory limitation on payments.' (Brazier *et al.*, 1998, pp. 72-73)

The report says of the Code of Practice that: 'It should seek to ensure that the interests of surrogates and commissioning couples are adequately protected and that all parties to an arrangement are clear about their expectations of each other'. (Brazier *et a/*, 1998, p. ii) However, it would not be legally binding on individuals: for them it would be merely an advisory code. Surrogate motherhood arrangements would remain legally unenforceable.

Obviously, it is desirable that the interest of surrogate mothers and commissioning parents are protected and it is very important that all parties to the agreement are clear about their reasonable expectations of each other. However, it is far from obvious that these interests would be well served by the implementation of Brazier's recommendations. In the absence of the legal enforceability of surrogate motherhood contracts, what are the reasonable expectations that one party can have of another? It is not clear what reasonably should be done or what it is reasonable to expect actually will be done.

It is said by the team that their proposed Code of Practice: '... should confirm that the welfare of the child to be born must be the paramount concern of all those involved in any surrogacy arrangement[1]. (Brazier *et al.*, 1998, p. ii) This is the language of the pulpit or the political rostrum rather than of the lectern or the study. Why should the interests of such children be paramount? Why should the interests of any particular category of people be paramount? In deciding whether or not, say, to join the Euro-zone, would one say that the interests of children should be paramount? Let us hope not. Children, after all, are not children for long but their interests, like they, outlive their childhood. Closer to home, even in legal decisions concerning divorce, the interests of any children of the marriage are not and should not be paramount.

What about the interests of a person – who was once a child and perhaps, even, a child of a surrogate motherhood arrangement – who wants now to be or to use a surrogate mother? Suppose that a particular commissioning couple are denied a parental order with regard to a particular child (whose biological parents the couple might be) because the couple paid the child's carrying mother more than reasonable expenses. Is such a denial in the interest of the child concerned? Why would it be? How can such a draconian, punitive measure be shown to accord with the (empty-sounding) claim about the paramouncy of the interests of the child to be born?

What, too, about the interests of those who might have been born were it not for the restrictions on surrogate motherhood of the sort advocated by Brazier and her colleagues? We shall return to this point.

Rationale for Recommendations

According to the Brazier report: 'Payments to surrogate mothers should cover only genuine expenses associated with the pregnancy.... Additional payments should be prohibited in order to prevent surrogacy arrangements being entered into for financial benefit...'. (Brazier, *el al*, 1998, p. 71)

What is wrong with 'financial benefit'? What is wrong with financially benefiting from being a surrogate mother (whether or not one became a surrogate mother in order solely to benefit financially)? What do Brazier and her colleagues – whether rightly or wrongly – think is wrong with these things? The quintessence of the case of the Review Team in support of its recommendations is as follows:

'We find that payments to surrogate mothers, other than in recompense for genuine expenses, give rise to the following concerns. (1) Payments create a danger that women will give less than free and fully informed consent to act as a surrogate. (2) Payments risk the commodification of the child to be born (3) Payments contravene the social norms of our society that, just as bodily parts cannot be sold, nor can such intimate services.' (Brazier *et al.*, 1998, p. i)

There are several sorts of problems with this suggested *rationale.* (See McLachlan and Swales, 2000b and 200la) First of all, even were the three suggested reasons to be accepted as justified grounds of concern, it is far from clear that they support the particular policy recommendations which the Brazier Team make. Secondly, the suggested reasons for concern are not good ones. Thirdly, there are other relevant arguments and issues that are not considered. Let us look at these points in turn.

The Relevance of Brazier's Arguments

It is said in their suggested *rationale* that there is an objection to the carrying mother's benefiting financially from being a carrying mother. However, their recommendations do not directly relate to this. Their recommendations would make it more difficult for a commissioning couple to become the legal parents of the relevant carried children if they are truthful in and towards the courts. Were their recommendations to be accepted, carrying mothers could still benefit financially from carrying the child. Their recommendations would not criminalise nor, necessarily, otherwise prevent the occurrence of paid surrogate motherhood.

Even if the Brazier recommendations were put into effect, surrogate mothers no less than at present could have a financial motive for being a surrogate mother and commissioning couples could have a motive for paying them. The effect of the recommendations would be to give them a motive for lying about how much had been paid if more had been paid than authorised expenses. This would arise if the commissioning parents wanted a parental order and the carrying mother wanted them to be granted one. A carrying mother might have a motive for saying that more than expenses had been paid even if they had not been should she change her mind and want to keep the baby.

Although the recommendations of Brazier and her colleagues relate mostly to the activities of surrogate motherhood agencies, their suggested *rationale* does not mesh with their recommendations. Whether agents and agencies should be allowed to receive payments for and/or make a profit from the entrepreneurial business of liaising between commissioning couples and carrying mothers is one thing and whether carrying mothers should benefit financially from being surrogate mothers is quite another one.

The Soundness of Brazier's Arguments

Furthermore, that there is an objection, as they envisage it, to the carrying mother's benefiting financially from the provision of her services is not established by Brazier and her colleagues. Their arguments are not an advance on those of the Warnock Report: they are, to a large extent, a repetition of them. There is, for instance, the familiar claim that payment for surrogate motherhood is against the 'values' of the Brazier team and of a majority of the public. Particularly in a society of various 'cultures' and 'values', (although, perhaps all societies are such) this type of plea should be rejected. One cares not what Brazier's or Warnock's or any one else's 'values' are in this context: one wants to hear what their arguments are. After all, beliefs, practices and actions are not reasonable, good, correct or true because Brazier or some one else happens to 'value' them: rather, if beliefs, practices and actions are true, reasonable and/or virtuous, then one should value them highly whether one does or not. If such beliefs, practices and actions are not in accord with one's 'values', then one should try to ignore or change one's 'values'. (See McLachlan, 1979.) Similarly, what public opinion happens to be is not the only relevant issue: what should public opinion be? One often looks to the law to protect people from what public opinion happens, on some issues, to be.

The apposite question is not: what is public opinion at the moment? If it were, there are better ways of finding out than setting up commissions and teams like those of Warnock and of Brazier. It would be more appropriate to commission a polling organisation. In so far as 'public opinion' is relevant, the appropriate question is more like the following. What would public opinion be if its members were all able to take the required time and effort to ponder and weigh all the possibly pertinent considerations rationally and impartially? If the Warnock Commission and the Brazier Review Team were not trying to answer a question such as this, then it is difficult to see what the manifest function of such commissions and teams is.

The curious claim about the risks associated with the lure of financial gain melts into the familiar argument that commercial surrogate motherhood is, or can be, exploitative. In essence, this is the claim on the part of Brazier and her team that they know better than do potential commercial surrogate mothers – or some of them – what their best interests are and what risks it is wise for them to run. (See McLachlan and Swales, 2001a) Even if one agreed that women act unwisely, or sometimes do when they decide to be commercial surrogate mothers, one might want to resist the paternalistic impulse to intrude in the decision.

Brazier *et al.* (1998, p.45) say:

'... it is a fundamental belief in our society that children should not be viewed as commodities to be bought and sold .... Although a theoretical distinction can be made between payment for purchase of a child and payment for a potentially risky, time-consuming and uncomfortable service, in practice it is difficult to separate the two, and it remains the case that payment other than for genuine expenses constitutes a financial benefit for the surrogate mother.'

Whether or not it is a fundamental belief of our society or, rather, of many of the members of our society, it is true that babies should not be – and cannot rationally be – regarded as commodities. Babies cannot and should not be bought and sold. We would suggest that to distinguish between the intelligible notion of paying a woman for her services and the unintelligible notion of paying someone for a baby is not a difficult intellectual exercise. (See McLachlan and Swales, 2000a) However, the issue does not necessarily pivot around this distinction. In a commercial surrogate motherhood transaction, what is actually bought and sold? Perhaps nothing is bought and sold. At the very least, one can assert unequivocally that babies are not bought and sold.

There is often quite a difference between what people think that they have bought and what they have actually bought. There is often quite a difference between what people think they are selling and what they are actually selling. There can be differences too between what people buy and sell and what other people think and/or say that they have bought and sold. It is not always the case that: 'What you have got is what you have bought'. If, for instance, you pay ransom to a kidnapper for the return of your child, you have not thereby bought your child from the kidnapper. What, if anything, have you bought? Nothing at all. You have effected, we would say, but not bought, the child's freedom. Often, in the absence of specific contracts and court decisions, it cannot be said what, if anything, actually has been bought or sold. Someone, in a pub in Britain let us say, might offer you a slave for sale. If you gave the person money and you were given another person in return, then you would not thereby have become the owner of a slave: you would not have bought a slave nor the services of one. It would be a misrepresentation of the situation to say that you had done so, even that you had illegally done so.

That which can be bought and sold must be, in some sense or other, property. Not everything actually is property. (See McLachlan, 1997b.) Not everything can be bought and sold. Babies are not property and neither is parenthood. Babies cannot be bought or sold and neither can parenthood. Consider, for instance, houses. Houses, as property, can be bought and sold. The owner of a house has a particular cluster of rights and duties relative to that house. If someone buys the house from him or her, then there will be a flow of money from the buyer to the seller and a corresponding transfer of the cluster of rights and duties from the initial owner to the new owner. Property is a complex matter and it can take various forms. However, one might say that the buying and selling of commodities in general shows a similar pattern to house purchase. It is the transfer of rights and duties relative to them rather than the physical transfer of the commodities themselves which constitutes buying and selling. One can, obviously, buy commodities that one fails to receive and receive things that one has not bought.

Notice, too, that ownership can be transferred in ways other than by buying and selling: for instance, property can be transferred as a gift or it can be forfeited as, say, a fine.

Services as well as 'tangible things' can be bought and sold (or transferred as gifts). Concerning the buying and selling of, say, houses, one might well pay other people for services that they provide in the facilitation of the transaction – lawyers, estate agents and so forth. (Lawyers and estate agents might waive their fees.) However, there is a distinction between payment to them for the services they provide and payment for the purchase of houses.

Suppose that you give us money and, in return, we hand over to you a baby. This situation is quite unlike the buying and selling (or the giving as a gift) of property. No cluster of legal rights and duties pertaining to the baby is, as a consequence of our supposed transaction, transferred from us to you. You might have possession of, but you do not have ownership of, the baby. Babies are not commodities: they cannot be bought and sold (nor given away) as commodities. Babies are not property. Similarly parenthood is not purchasable (nor transferable by gift): it is, like the state of being married, a particular conferred legal status: it is not a form of property. Parents do not own their babies although they might own – and be able to sell – some things pertaining to them such as, say, privately taken photographs of them.

Even if babies were commodities, it does not follow that they legally could be and actually would be treated in the same ways that, for instance, inanimate commodities may be and are treated. To say that one owns something most certainly does not imply that one can do with it what one wants. (See McLachlan, 1997b) Ownership can involve severe duties and can carry with it, sometimes, rights only of a very restrictive sort. Cats and lumps of coal can be commodities. It does not follow that owners of cats and lumps of coal are allowed to do with them what they will, nor that they actually do treat cats and lumps of coal the same way in all respects.

It is not necessarily wrong to treat babies, in some respects, in the same way that we treat commodities. It depends on the ways and the respects. While it would be wrong to treat babies in all respects in the ways in which some commodities might, not inappropriately, be treated, it is not wrong to treat babies in some respects as some or even all commodities might, not inappropriately, be treated. For instance, some commodities, especially expensive ones, are cleaned, cherished and insured. It is not wrong to clean, cherish and insure babies.

The Comprehensiveness of Brazier *et al.*'s arguments: Feminism; Human Rights; and Social Exclusion

The Brazier report, like the Warnock one before it, is, in its discussion of surrogate motherhood, not sufficiently comprehensive: far from all the relevant arguments are discussed.

According to, for instance, Anderson, there is a strong feminist case for prohibiting commercial surrogate agreements and agencies. She says that: 'While contract pregnancy brings financial rewards to a few women, it reinforces gendered relations of inequality and stereotypes that undermine the status of women in general'. (Anderson, 1993, p. 185) She says:

'Critics of contract pregnancy argue that it reinforces negative stereotypes of women that prevent them gaining equality with men. It reinforces the gendered division of labor that keeps women subordinate to men by confining them to domestic work. It also supports the sexist view of women as primarily valuable for providing shelter for the genetic offspring of men.' (Anderson, 1993, p. 182)

Tong, too, speaks powerfully from a feminist position against surrogate motherhood, especially commercial surrogate motherhood although she makes it clear that there is also a strong feminist case in support of surrogate motherhood including commercial surrogate motherhood. (See Tong, 1997, pp. 199-212)

Which of the feminist arguments are good ones and which are weak? Which feminist arguments should be accepted and why should they be accepted? The Brazier Report, like the Warnock one before it, does not say. This is a weakness in it. We do not necessarily accept Anderson's arguments but in what is supposed to be a review of the law and public policy concerning surrogate motherhood, they should be, in our view, considered. If they are dismissed as a reason for supporting legislation then that they are dismissed, and why they are dismissed, should be indicated. Why what is done as well as what is done is important.

The Brazier Report is also lacking in comprehensiveness in its failure to consider surrogate motherhood in relation to debates about (so-called) human rights. We are not very comfortable with the notion of a 'human right' to procreate. It is, rather, our view that whether or not people have a 'right' to procreate – whether or not a 'human right' – there is a strong case for allowing them to do so and even, often, for helping them to do so unless there are particularly powerful contrary arguments. One does not require a human right to X in order for it to be wise to allow the doing of X to be legal. Nonetheless, the arguments about surrogate motherhood and human rights need, in any comprehensive analysis of the issues concerning surrogate motherhood, to be addressed and weighed. (See, for instance Robertson, 1983; Singer and Wells, 1985; Gostin, 1988; Kymlicka, 1991; and Gostin, 2001)

Harris (2000, p. 33) says:

'The Brazier Report and the HFE Act, violate, or recommend violations, not only of our shared morality, which attaches great importance to choice in matters of procreation, but of the right to found a family, a right or liberty protected by Article 16 of the Universal Declaration of Human Rights and article 12 of the European Convention on Human Rights.'

Whether or not this criticism is justified, that the Brazier Report is open to it is noteworthy.

People are sometimes said – by dint of stipulative definition – to be in 'poverty' if they lack the resources to obtain the sorts of goods and services that are typically enjoyed by their fellow citizens. (See Townsend, 1984, McLachlan, 1983 and 1986 and Veit Wilson, 1986) It is, often, in a similar spirit that policymakers and policy-formulators advocate social inclusion rather than its opposite. To have children and children that are thought of as 'one's own' is a very common aspiration and attainment. Those who have the aspiration without the attainment can be thought of as being victims of 'social exclusion' of a sort and of a sort that is significant and hurtful to them. In a sense, childless couples who want the services of commercial surrogate mothers are doubly excluded: they are excluded by the Brazier Report from the category of those whose exclusion is talked of as 'social exclusion' and considered worthy of rectification. They merit, in our view, more sympathy – constructive sympathy – and consideration than the Brazier Report gives to them and their plight.

The Moral Status of the Unborn

Among the anomalies and confusions in the Brazier Report, Harris has recently noted the following. It is claimed simultaneously in the

Report both that the 'welfare of the child' is paramount and that there should be regulations such that that various children who might otherwise be born as a result of commercial surrogate motherhood will not be born. Something seems to have gone wrong here. As Harris (2000, p. 33) says:

'To give the "highest priority ... to the welfare of the child to be born" is always to let that child come into existence, unless existence overall will be a burden rather than a benefit. Wherever that child's life, despite predictable suboptimalities, will be thoroughly worth living, then it cannot be that child's interest which justify any decisions or regulations which would deny it opportunities for existence.'

Harris, it seems to us, is correct here (although, unlike Harris, we do not subscribe to the view that the welfare of such children should be 'paramount'.) We have written elsewhere, in connection with commercial surrogate motherhood:

'After all, it is surely better to be born with one's dignity violated than not to be born at all. If the only way that a particular person could be born is through becoming an object of barter then no obvious favour is being done to that person by failing to allow him to become an object of barter.' (McLachlan and Swales, 2000b, p. 119)

Brazier and her colleagues come to their particular anomalous position by way of the assumption – since explicitly indicated by Campbell in defence of the report – that only people who have bodies which are currently alive have moral rights and/or are due moral consideration from those who do have such live bodies. (See Campbell, 2000) They discuss the situation where, because of legal disallowment, a surrogate motherhood arrangement that would have taken place does not take place and, consequently, someone who might have been born is not born. They say: '... there is no child who suffers the loss or to whom we or the parents have moral obligations'. (Brazier *et al.*, p. 36) This is a dubious claim to make. We would say that the person whose body might have been carried by the surrogate mother can be the bearer or rights and the object of obligations. (See McLachlan, 1977, 2002a and 2002b)

The view is not self-evidently correct that only people who have bodies that are currently alive have moral rights and/or are due moral consideration. It is asserted rather than argued for by Brazier *et al.* It is particularly unfortunate that such a view should be presented in a report to Health Ministers since there is no reason why this particular view should be given preferred political status. It is presented in the report as if it were a discovery from the deliberations of its members when it is nothing of the sort. The tone and content of the Brazier Report are maddening and lead one to wonder what sort of a thing a Report to Health Ministers is supposed, by its compilers, to be.

Conclusion

We have not resolved the debate about what the law and public policy should be regarding surrogate motherhood and neither have we tried to. We have, however, shown that the present situation requires to be reconsidered and that the argumentation of the Brazier report, no less than that of the Warnock report, is unsatisfactory.

*By Hugh V McLachlan and J. Kim Swales, *Human Reproduction and Genetic Ethics*, Vol. 11, No. 1, 2005, pp. 12-23.

References

Anderson, Elizabeth, 1993, *Value in Ethics and Economics,* Harvard University Press/The MIT Press.

Brazier, Margaret, Campbell, Alastair and Golombok, Susan, 1998, *Surrogacy: Review for Health Ministers of Current Arrangements for Payments and Regulations; Report of the Review Team,* Cm 4068.

Campbell, Alastair, V., 2000, 'Surrogacy, Rights and Duties: A Partial Commentary', *Health Care Analysis,* Vol. 8, No. 1, pp. 35-40.

Freeman, M., 1989, 'Is Surrogacy Exploitative?' in *Legal Issues in Human Reproduction,* Sheila McLean, (editor), Aldershot, Gower.

Galbraith, Mhairi, McLachlan, Hugh V. and Swales, J. Kim (2005) 'Commercial Surrogacy Agencies: A Transactions Costs Approach,' *Health Care Analysis*, Vol.13, No.1.

Gostin, L., 1988, 'A Civil Liberties Analysis of Surrogacy Arrangements', *Law, Medicine and Health Care,* Vol. 16, pp. 7-17.

Gostin, L., 2001, 'Surrogacy From the Perspectives of Economic and Civil Liberties', *The Journal of Contemporary Health Law and Policy,* Vol. 17, pp. 429-431.

Harris, John, 2000, The Welfare of the Child', *Health Care Analysis,* Vol. 8, No. 1, pp. 27-34.

Kymlicka, Will, 1991, 'Re-thinking the Family: Review of Okin's Justice, Gender and the Family', *Philosophy and Public Affairs,* Vol. 20, pp. 77-97.

McHale, Jean and Fox, Marie with Murphy, John, 1999, *Health Care*

Law: Text, Cases and Materials, Sweet and Maxwell, London.
McLachlan Hugh V., 1977, 'Must We Accept Either the Conservative or the Liberal View on Abortion?', *Analysis,* Vol. 37, No. 4, pp. 197-204.
McLachlan, Hugh V., 1979, The Is/Ought Question: A Needless Controversy', *Journal of the British Society for Phenomenology,* Vol. 10, No. 2, pp. 134-137.
McLachlan, Hugh V., 1983, Townsend and the Concept of "Poverty"', *Social Policy and Administration,* Vol. 17, No. 2, pp. 97-105.
McLachlan, Hugh V., 1986, 'Concepts of Poverty and Deprivation', *Journal of Social Policy,* Vol. 15, No. 4, pp. 499-501.
McLachlan, Hugh V., 1993, 'Warnock and Research on Human Embryos: A Case for a Reappraisal of the Fertilisation and Embryology Act (1990)', *International Journal of Sociology and Social Policy,* Vol. 13, Nos. 5/6, pp. 110-119.
McLachlan, Hugh V., 1997a, 'Defending Commercial Surrogate Motherhood Against Van Niekerk and Van Zyl, *Journal of Medical Ethics,* Vol. 23, No. 6, pp. 344-348.
McLachlan, Hugh V., 1997b, 'Bodies, Rights and Abortion', *Journal of Medical Ethics,* Vol. 23, No. 3, pp. 176-180.
McLachlan, Hugh V., 2002a, 'Bodies, Persons and Research on Human Embryos', *Human Reproduction and Genetic Ethics,* Vol. 8, No. 1, pp. 4-6.
McLachlan, Hugh V., 2002b, 'Persons and Their Bodies: How We Should Think About Human Embryos', *Health Care Analysis,* Vol. 10, No. 2.
McLachlan, Hugh V. and Swales, J. Kim, 2000a, 'Babies, Child Bearers and Commodification: Anderson, Brazier *et al.* and the Political Economy of Commercial Surrogate Motherhood', *Health Care Analysis,* Vol. 8, No 1, pp. 1-18.
McLachlan, Hugh V. and Swales, J. Kim, 2000b, 'Scotland, the Church and Surrogate Motherhood', *Scottish Affairs,* No. 32, Summer, pp. 110-123.
McLachlan, Hugh V. and Swales, J. Kim, 2001a, 'Exploitation and Commercial Surrogate Motherhood', *Human Reproduction and Genetic Ethics,* Vol. 7, No. 1, pp. 8-14.
McLachlan, Hugh V. and Swales, J. Kim, 2001b, 'Surrogate Motherhood, Rights and Duties: A Reply to Campbell', *Health Care Analysis,* Vol. 9, No. 1. pp. 101-107.
Robertson, John, 1983, *Surrogate Mothers: Not so Novel after All,* Hastings Centre Report, October, pp. 28-34.

Singer, Peter and Wells, Deane, 1985, *Making Babies: The New Science and Ethics of Contraception,* New York, Charles Scribner's Sons.

Tong, Rosemary, 1997, *Feminist Approaches to Bioethics,* Westview Press, Oxford.

Townsend, Peter, 1984, 'A Rejoinder on Poverty', *Social Policy and Administration,* Vol. 18, No. 2, pp. 165-167.

Veit-Wilson, John, 'Paradigms of Poverty: A Rehabilitation of B.S. Rowntree', *Journal of Social Policy,* Vol. 5, No. 1, pp. 69-99.

Warnock, Mary, (Chairman), 1984. *Report of the Committee of Inquiry into Human Fertilisation and Embryology,* H.M.S.O., London, Cmnd. 9314. Reprinted in Warnock, 1985.

Warnock, Mary, 1985, *A Question of Life: The Warnock Report on Human Fertilisation and Embryology,* Basil Blackwell, Oxford.

Wertheimer, Alan, 1996, *Exploitation,* Princeton University Press, Princeton.

Altruism and Blood Donation

Chapter Fifteen

The Unpaid Donation of Blood and Altruism: a Comment on Keown*

Abstract

In line with article 3.4 of EC directive 89/381, Keown has presented an ethical case in support of the policy of voluntary, unpaid donation of blood. Although no doubt is cast on the desirability of the policy, that part of Keown's argument which pertains to the suggested laudability of altruism and of its encouragement by social policy is examined and shown to be dubious.

Introduction

Keown presents "an ethical case in favour of voluntary, unpaid donation [of blood and plasma]. It comprises five arguments".[1] I shall discuss and strongly disagree with one of these arguments, the one about "altruism and social solidarity". Keown's claim that: "There would appear to be at least five sound reasons for discouraging, as a matter of social policy, paid donation of blood and plasma" is, I shall suggest, a dubious one.[2]

That there is a sound non-ethical case for favouring this system of blood and plasma collection – it is, for instance, cheaper for the taxpayer and likely to be safer than alternative systems -and that this case suffices to establish a preference for it I do not doubt.

Keown on altruism and blood donation

Keown writes:

"A major argument for exclusive reliance on unpaid donation is that, unlike paid donation, it promotes altruism and social solidarity. Titmuss, in his landmark study of blood donation and social policy, wrote that his study was essentially about 'the role of altruism in modern society'."[3]

Keown agrees with Singer's view "... that altruism is a virtue which increases the more it is practised" and says that: "The old maxim that an act tends to become a habit and a habit tends to form a character seems apt." [4]

The following quotation from Murray is presented with approval by Keown:

"'Gifts to strangers affirm the solidarity of the community over and above the depersonalizing, alienating forces of mass society and market relations. They signal that self-interest is not the only significant human motivation. And they express the moral belief that it is good to minister to fundamental human needs, needs for food, health care and shelter.... These universal needs irrevocably tie us together in a community of needs, with a shared desire to satisfy them, and see them satisfied in others'."[5]

According to Keown:

"An individual who acts altruistically tends thereby to develop an altruistic *character* and becomes more rather than less disposed to act altruistically. It is obvious too that the same holds in relation to the person who performs selfish acts: the person who (say) steals other people's property tends thereby to develop a rapacious character.... In short, acts of altruism promote further acts of altruism in that they tend to reinforce altruistic dispositions."[6]

Against altruism or, at least, the encouragement of it

Keown states or seems to imply something like the following propositions:

(i) Non-paid voluntary blood donation is, because it is voluntary and unpaid, altruistic;

(ii) Altruism in general is a particularly good thing; and

(iii) Social policy should be formulated to encourage altruism because altruism is a particularly good thing.

Each of the claims is contentious.

Consider, first of all,(i). When people submit contributions to, say, the *Journal of Medical Ethics,* their actions are voluntary and unpaid: does it follow from this that they are altruistic? I do not see that it does. The writing and offering for consideration for publication of such papers might be but need not be altruistic. Not all actions are either done for the sake of money or are altruistic. Some are both. Some are neither. Those which are altruistic are not always morally more laudable than the rest. Even when actions are morally laudable, it is not always appropriate that, through the formulation of social policy, they and/or the motivation which provoked them be given encouragement by the state.

In relation to (ii) and (iii), consider the following passage.

"The child sat by and watched its progress with a troubled mind. Regardless of the run of luck, and mindful only of the desperate passion which had its hold upon her grandfather, losses and gains were to her alike. Exulting in some brief triumph, or cast down by a defeat, there he sat so wild and restless, so feverishly and intensely anxious, so terribly eager, so ravenous for the paltry stakes, that she could have almost borne better to see him dead. And yet she was the innocent cause of all this torture, and he, gambling with such a savage thirst for gain as the most insatiable gambler never felt, had not one selfish thought!"[7]

The grandfather of little Nell, from *The Old Curiosity Shop* here, has not one selfish thought. He is an altruist. He is gambling – for money, of course, but – for the sake of his granddaughter. His actions, although altruistic – the prelude, he hopes, to the gift to little Nell of the money thereby gained – are wrong. They are vicious in the sense of being in the character of a vice. It is certain that his altruistic action should not be encouraged! The less this particular manifestation of altruism is practised the better.

Keown is making and suggesting false dichotomies. Actions can be altruistic and wrong and worthy of discouragement. They can also be altruistic and done for money. Furthermore, merely because an action was done for the sake of money does not mean nor imply that the action is wrong nor, necessarily, in any respect morally dubious even although such actions can be, like some particular altruistic actions, very wrong. They can also be worthy of discouragement by the state, sometimes, as well as by private moral agents.

It is manifest that good outcomes can result from the self-interested pursuit of money. For instance, Dickens's *The Old Curiosity Shop*, which was written for money, is, even allowing for the appalling over-sentimentalisation of Nell's death, more worthy in all respects which I can think of than many other examples of prose which were not written for monetary gain, including the one you are now reading, and than many which were written, let us allow, for altruistic reasons such as, say, *The Communist Manifesto* and Titmuss's *The Gift Relationship*.

Altruism can and often does produce havoc. Guy Fawkes and the other wretched gunpowder conspirators were not motivated by monetary considerations. They would probably have done more good and risked the production of less harm if they had been. Often, altruism results in extremely wicked actions because people can, wrongly, be prepared to do for other people things which they would, rightly, be too ashamed to do solely for themselves. The recent suicide bombers in Israel, who killed over a dozen bystanders in a crowded market-place and injured many more were not – or possibly were not – lacking in altruism. However, altruism is no more inherently good than the pursuit of monetary gain is inherently bad. Notice too that it is to paid policemen and paid soldiers rather than to enthusiastic and altruistic amateurs that we look for protection from such violent and, often, woefully non-self-regarding people.

Some people might want to say here – although I for one can resist this temptation – that such seemingly altruistic acts as terroristic ones are not, when properly interpreted, truly altruistic at all but, of course, this would invite the response that the same thing could be said about unpaid blood donation.

Altruism can be good in some contexts and can be bad in others. It can have good effects as well as bad effects. It can be done for good motives as well as bad ones: altruistic motives are not always good; self-interested motives – and these are not always "selfish" ones – are not always bad. Furthermore, there is no convincing *a priori* case for expecting altruistic motives and actions to be good or self-interested ones to be bad. Social policy should be no more geared in general towards the fostering of altruism rather than self-interest, including that which is related to pecuniary gain.

Suppose, for instance, that you were to marry someone purely for altruistic reasons. Such an action with such a motivation would be rotten. It would be appallingly bad. It would, I think, be even worse than marrying someone purely for financial gain.

Conclusion

I do not know whether altruism in the abstract and in general can be nurtured – perhaps this is a psychological rather than a philosophical issue – but, if it can be, I see – as a philosophico-ethical matter – no reason why such altruism rather than, say, the pursuit of self-interested monetary gain should be encouraged by the state or by any other agency or person.

If the altruistic donation of blood is such an unreservedly good thing, then why stop at the donation of a pint? Why not give two pints, or three, or …? Why not, in an act of altruistic suicide, donate the whole lot? The answer, of course, is that altruism untempered is not a good thing. Altruism is a good thing only in the context of, amongst other things, the pursuit of self-interest and the acquisition of money.

Vitamin C can be good for us. I do not think that it necessarily follows from that that politicians and/or "social-policy makers" should encourage us to consume vitamin C. Manifestly, it does not follow that they should encourage us not to eat food which does not contain vitamin C. They should not encourage us to eat only vitamin C.

Analogously, to lead a good life, in all senses of "goodness", we need a healthy, balanced diet of motives and actions, which includes altruistic and non-altruistic actions, self-interested and non-self-interested actions, actions performed for money and actions which are not performed for money and ones which are a combination of two or more of these sorts. The idea that "social policy" should be formulated in order to encourage one rather than another of these types of motives and actions is misguided. It seems to me to be misplaced sentimentality, masquerading as moral sensitivity.

*By Hugh V McLachlan from the *Journal of Medical Ethics*, 1998, Vol. 24, No. 4, pp. 252-254. Reproduced with permission from the BMJ publishing group.

References

(1) Keown J. The gift of blood in Europe: an ethical defence of EC directive 89/381. *Journal of Medical Ethics* 1997; 23: 96-100.
(2) See reference 1:99.
(3) See reference 1:96.
(4) See reference 1:97-98.
(5) See reference 1:97.
(6) See reference 1:98
(7) Dickens C. *The old curiosity shop*. London and Glasgow, Collins, 1992:213.

Chapter Sixteen

Altruism, Blood Donation and Public Policy: A Reply to Keown*

Abstract

This is a continuation of and a development of a debate between John Keown and me. The issue discussed is whether, in Britain, an unpaid system of blood donation promotes and is justified by its promotion of altruism. Doubt is cast on the notions that public policies can, and, if they can, that they should, be aimed at the promotion and expression of altruism rather than of self-interest, especially that of a mercenary sort. Reflections upon President Kennedy's proposition, introduced into the debate by Keown, that we should ask not what our country can do for us but what we can do for our country is pivotal to this casting of doubt. A case is made for suggesting that advocacy along the lines which Keown presents of an exclusive reliance on a voluntary, unpaid system of blood donation encourages inappropriate attitudes towards the provision of health care. Perhaps, it is suggested, and the suggestion represents, on my part, a change of mind as a consequence of the debate, a dual system of blood provision might be preferable.

Introduction

According to Keown, I have misinterpreted his views on altruism and blood donation and have presented my own case unclearly.1-3 I will deal with both of these objections of Keown's, question his account of the relationship between particular public policies and the promotion of altruism, and then indicate how reflection on his thoughts is leading me to change my mind, not about the nature of altruism and public policy, but about the desirability of an exclusive reliance upon a system of voluntary, unpaid blood donation.

The interpretation of what Keown wrote

Keown writes:

"Dr McLachlan proceeds to state that not all altruistically motivated acts are morally superior to non-altruistically motivated acts and that it is not always appropriate for the state to encourage altruism. Again, I nowhere suggest the contrary." [4]

In his original article, he says the following, which did and still does suggest to me the contrary:

"A major argument for exclusive reliance on unpaid donation is that, unlike paid donation, it promotes altruism and social solidarity."[5]

In his reply, he says things which suggest to me the contrary, such as the following:

"Surely unselfishness is something that a community should (or at the very least may) encourage among its members, both in the interests of its individual members and the community as a whole? Surely any community, whether a family, college, or state, is enriched by the altruism of its members, by their willingness to have regard to the interests of others and act unselfishly? And for the state to promote such altruism and provide means for its expression, whether by encouraging, through its system of taxation, donations of money to charitable causes, or through its health system, donations of blood to others in need, is not only defensible but commendable." [4]

Whether or not Keown here means to state that altruism should, in the abstract, be encouraged by the state, it seems to me that what he says invites or at least suggest that interpretation. His quotations, with obvious approval, from the work of Titmuss, who, in relation to social policy, is the champion of altruism, also suggest that this interpretation is a fair one.

Keown gives no textual support for his attack on my interpretation of what he wrote (as opposed, say, to what he believes or to what he meant to say). His attack on me and defence of himself amounts to the argument that I attributed to him a position which could not consistently or rationally be held. The argument, although true when thus phrased, is not much of an attack on me or of a defence of himself. I did and do claim that such a position is suggested by what he wrote. Hence, I am not at all impressed when Keown says: "... to be accused by Dr McLachlan of making and suggesting false dichotomies is remarkable".[6] It is not remarkable at all.

Note that in his reply to my comment upon him, Keown persists in making and suggesting false dichotomies, as in the two following sentences:

"Was President Kennedy wrong when he said that we should not ask what our country can do for us, but what we can do for our country? Yet Dr McLachlan states that he sees no reason why the state should encourage altruism over the 'self – interested' pursuit of money." [4]

I can see no reason "why the state should encourage altruism over the 'self-interested' pursuit of money" because Keown, despite his intention and claims, has provided none. Keown has provided none because, I suspect, there is none. Again, he gives the appearance of presenting as a dichotomy altruism, as if it were on the one hand, and the accepting of money, as if it were on the other. Why does Keown put "self-interested" in quotation marks? Are they meant to be scare quotations marks?

This leads to the matter of my views on blood donation and altruism as expressed in my comment.

Blood donation, altruism and public policy

I wrote that I was in favour of the present system of unpaid blood donation. There are good reasons for that system but the promotion of altruism, in the abstract – whether or not it can be so promoted – is not, in my view, one of them.

Actions can be self-interested and, even, involve the acquisition of money and also be altruistic. It is misleading to suggest a dichotomy of altruism and self-interest.

Neither altruism nor self-interest in the abstract should be – if they can be – fostered by the state. Altruism in the abstract is no better or worse than self-interest in the abstract. Both are required for a balanced individual and a healthy society and state. Both can lead to good consequences in some circumstances and bad ones in others. Both can be, in some circumstances good motives for actions and in some circumstances bad motives. I am not sure that the encouragement of any sort of attitudes rather than the encouragement of particular sorts of actions and behaviour is the proper business of the state. Some particular manifestations of self-interest, including that directed towards the acquisition of money, should be encouraged by the state, some should be allowed by the state and some should be prohibited by the state. The same can be said of manifestations of altruism.

The idea is misguided, in my view, that it is desirable for social policy to be geared towards, in the abstract and in general, the promotion of altruism. The idea is mistaken too that, were there to be a makeable choice, social policies should be preferred which provoke and/or are provoked by altruism rather than those which provoke and/or are provoked by self-interest.

My views on altruism might be clarified, if clarification is required, and developed, possibly, by my responding to Keown's jibe about Kennedy.

Altruism, self-interest and President Kennedy

Was Kennedy wrong when he said what Keown said he said? Yes he was, or would have been were he to have been speaking, when he did, as a philosopher rather than as a politician. We should not ask what we can do for our country rather than what our country can do for us. We should ask both these (and other related) questions but neither question carries moral priority over the other.

If membership of a particular country involved nothing but self-sacrifice from its members then it would not be much of a country and its members should think about altering or abandoning it. Indeed, were not Kennedy's British ancestors very keen to ask what precisely their country did for them? To say, for instance, "No taxation without representation" is to be – and rightly to be – very conscious of the question: "What does my country do for me?". If President Kennedy had been around as a politician at the time of the Boston Tea Party, would he have said to his fellow British-Americans: "Ask not what Britain can do for you but, rather, what you can do for Britain?" I doubt it.

Notice that Kennedy does not say that we should ask what we can do for our country rather than what we can and should do for ourselves. Kennedy does not say that we should be wary about the acquisition of money. If Kennedy is implying a dichotomy, then, despite what Keown night think or lead the reader to think, it is a different dichotomy from the one which Keown suggests. Kennedy is not saying here – did he say it any where else? – that the state, if faced with the choice, should encourage altruism over the self-interested pursuit of money. (Is Keown trying to suggest that Kennedy was, despite all appearances, some sort of a socialist?) In any case, it is one thing for citizens to ask what they can and should do for their country, it is another thing for the state to have social policies about it. Kennedy does not say that one should ask what one should do for one's country rather than earn money for one's self. What, in any case, should one do for one's country? I would say, and I imagine that President Kennedy would have agreed, that what we can and should do for our country is to earn enough money to meet the needs of our selves and our families so that we are able, when we are required to do so, to act altruistically towards others and so that we are not an avoidable drain on the altruism and benevolence of others. The altruism of other people is not like a muscle which they have and of which the exercise should be encouraged in order to make it more powerful. It is a scarce resource which should be tapped, if at all, gingerly.

Due regard to our own interests and, even, to our own wallets is a proper and sometimes an obligatory manifestation of our altruism. What, perhaps, we should do for our country, for our families and ourselves is get a paying job. If we cannot get a paying job then, perhaps, in some circumstances, we should, if we can, sell our blood or other renewable bodily parts and services.

Public policy and the promotion of altruism

That public policies in general can, and that the particular policies of voluntary, unpaid blood donation and of tax relief on donations to charity actually do, foster altruism in general is claimed but not proved by Keown. The claims, which I take to be psychological and, possibly, sociological rather than philosophical ones might well be true but they are not obviously true.

When, say, the state gives tax relief for donations to charity, I am not sure whether this is a wise policy. If it is justifiable, then it is justifiable – not as the promotion of altruism in general and as such but – as the encouragement of donations to charity, whatever might be the motivation of the donators.

Incidentally, I know of no British social policy, although there might be plenty, which was justified by the politicians who promoted it on, or largely on, the grounds that it promoted, in the abstract, altruism. Is there any?

Keown's views on the encouragement of the existence and expression of altruism by way of public policies are interesting but contentious. They provoke in me this reflection: the more the state makes it attractive or not unattractive to give to charities through, say, tax incentives, the more it encourages the giving to charities but the less, one might say, it gives scope for the altruism involved of the givers. If, say, those who gave to charities were, by order of the government, to be severely flogged, then less would be given to charities but that which was given – at least by non-masochists – might be more altruistically provided.

Such public policies as Keown mentions need not make people any more or less selfish although they might render more or less selfish the performance of particular actions. Tax relief on donations to charities increases donations to charities when it does, not by encouraging nor providing a means of expression of altruism (of which there is not a shortage), but by reducing the motivational force of self-regard which, in this particular instance, pulls in the other direction from altruism. Given a particular blend and strengths of self-regarding, altruistic and other motives – which blend and strengths remain unaffected by the policy measure – what tax relief on donations to charity does, as a policy of severely flogging givers to charity would do, is to alter the attractiveness to the potential givers of giving to charity. Thus, a policy which increased donations to charity would be a quite different sort from one – whatever that might be – which would increase altruism. Similarly, a policy which encouraged voluntary, unpaid blood donation might or might not encourage and promote altruism.

A system of compulsory, unpaid blood donation or voluntary, paid blood donation might, without resulting in a reduction of altruism, produce more blood. If those who are now prepared to donate blood when there is no payment involved became unwilling to do so when money changed hands, then, despite what Keown suggests, one might think that such people were motivated to give blood by vainglory rather than by altruism.

It is possible that through the unpaid donating of their blood, people thereby strengthen their tastes for other altruistic and charitable actions. On the other hand, it is possible that they do not. It is possible too that the time and effort involved in the donation of blood might be better spent in some other altruistic and charitable pursuits at the expense of which – in the sense of the opportunity cost – the blood is donated.

It is not clear how public policies would promote or do the opposite to altruism and it is far from obvious that such policies should be directed towards the promotion of altruism. Not only can one envisage societies and economies which persist on the basis of self-interest with altruism being required to plug the gaps, as it were, history provides numerous examples of them. Societies and economies which persist on the basis of altruism with self-interest plugging the gaps are not only, at least for non-Marxists, difficult to envisage but also, history provides no examples of industrialised ones. Perhaps in this sense self-interest is more important than altruism, at least with regard to public and social policies and for impersonal rather than intimate, face-to-face relationships. Altruism, despite what Keown seems to me to suggest, is not something which should be maximised; and, furthermore, the mix of altruism and self-interest which is optimal for, say, to use his examples, a family or a college, need not be optimal for a community or for a society or for a state.

Conclusion

I was in favour of a system of voluntary, unpaid blood donation on the grounds that there are good (non-ethical) reasons for the adoption of such a system in, say, contemporary Britain although not necessarily in all other places: it provides good blood and blood that is cheap to the tax-payer. However, my views in this matter are, I think, in a state of flux. I feel myself being attracted to the view that there should be, in Britain, a dual system of blood donation or, at least, that there should be no state discouragement of the emergence and operation of one.

If people want to give their blood for no payment and agents and agencies of the National Health Service and other lawful people and bodies want to take it from them that is fine. Fine too, I think, it would be if people wanted to sell their blood and other lawful people and bodies wanted to buy it from them.

I suspect that it might be preferable for the state to allow the existence of both systems of blood acquisition. It might be preferable for the following reasons. It is one thing to support an exclusively voluntary and unpaid system of blood donation for non-ethical reasons. It might be another to support it, as Keown does, on ethical grounds, as part of the advocacy of altruism. The latter approach – as Keown's reply and the re-reading of his original article leads me to suspect – can have the unfortunate consequence of encouraging two inappropriate attitudes towards the provision of health care and related services.

How such services should be provided and distributed in contemporary Britain is – like the matter of how other crucially important things like food and books should be provided and distributed – fundamentally an economic issue, which can have ethical implications. It is this and is better thought of as this, than as being fundamentally an ethical issue, which might have economic implications. Advocacy of unpaid blood donation on ethical grounds might encourage the latter inappropriate view of the matter.

Similarly, the view might be encouraged that it is better freely to give and receive rather than to buy and sell and that it is wrong to buy and sell body parts and bodily services or, at least, that it is morally preferable to donate them freely. Such a view is, I think, not only false but it can have, when acted upon, bad consequences. An instance of this is the allowing, in Britain, of surrogate motherhood where there is no payment made by the commissioning couple to the surrogate mother but the disallowing of commercial surrogate motherhood.

There are advantages and disadvantages of getting, say, a fitted kitchen provided for you by enthusiastic, kind-hearted friends. There are advantages and disadvantages of paying a professional kitchen-fitter to fit your kitchen: it is more expensive but with commercial kitchen-fitting, once the job is done you can quietly and effectively sever all ties with the kitchen-fitter if you are happy with the service you have received, and live the rest of you life without his/her intrusive presence; if you are not happy then you have the possibility of legal redress. So too with surrogate motherhood. There are advantages and disadvantages of an unpaid system and advantages and disadvantages of a commercial system. Let both systems exist, as with the fitting of kitchens – and let the potential users decide which system they prefer to use. So too, I suspect, it should be with blood.

Keown writes in his reply to me:

"... if paid donation were introduced, why would this not encourage many to donate out of purely selfish motives, radically transforming the entire culture the blood donation system in the process?"[4]

Notice that in my comment, I did not advocate payment for blood donation: I was not even think-about doing so when I wrote it. After further reflection on Keown 's views, I think I might do so now.

Some people might fit kitchens out of purely selfish motives. That does not suggest to me that the commercial fitting of kitchens should be discouraged or disallowed. People might write, publish or sell books out of purely selfish motives but that is not much of a reason for disfavouring the availability of commercially produced and supplied books. If some people were to sell their blood purely for selfish reasons, so what? For the reasons stated concerning the two inappropriate attitudes towards health-care provision, I would not be unhappy to see the culture of the blood transfusion system – indeed the entire, peculiarly British way of thinking about the provision and distribution of health-care services – transformed.

*By Hugh V McLachlan, from the *Journal of Medical Ethics*, 1999, Vol. 25, No. 6, pp. 532-536. Reproduced with permission from the BMJ publishing group.

References

(1) Keown J. The gift of blood in Europe: an ethical defence of EC directive 89/381. *Journal of Medical Ethics* 1997; 23: 96-100.
(2) Keown J. A Reply to McLachlan. *Journal of Medical Ethics.* 1998;24:255-6/
(3) McLachlan HV The unpaid donation of blood and altruism: a comment on Keown. *Journal of Medical Ethics* 1998; 24:252-4.
(4) See reference 2:256.
(5) See reference 1:96
(6) See reference 2:255.

Health and Health Care – Justice, Rights and Equality

Chapter Seventeen

A Drunk Driver, a Sober Pedestrian and the Allocation of Tragically Scarce and Indivisible Emergency Hospital Treatment*

Abstract

Le Grand describes a situation where a drunk driver, who has medical insurance, is the cause of an accident in which he and a sober pedestrian, who has no medical insurance, are both equally and seriously injured. At the private hospital to which they are both taken, there is available emergency treatment for one of them only. Who should receive it? The issues raised by Le Grand's example are shown to be more interesting, more complex and less clear-cut than Le Grand suggests and implies. In particular, it is not the case that, unequivocally, the drunkenness of the driver establishes that the pedestrian rather than he should be treated nor that, unequivocally, the driver's possession of health insurance is morally irrelevant.

Key words: equality, fairness, justice, private health care, rights

Introduction

'Nor do I in any way approve of the modern sympathy with invalids. I consider it morbid. Illness of any kind is hardly a thing to be encouraged in others. Health is the primary duty of life. I am always telling that to your poor uncle ...' Lady Bracknell in *The Importance of Being Ernest* by Oscar Wilde.

Julian Le Grand presents an extremely interesting envisaged situation which raises important questions concerning the economics, politics and ethics of health care provision. He also suggests answers to some of these questions. We shall continue the discussion of these questions and answers (McLachlan, 1995).

The Accident and its Aftermath

He sets the scene as follows:

'Late at night, a car being driven at speed mounts the pavement and hits a pedestrian out walking her dog. The car then crashes into a wall. Both driver and the pedestrian are critically injured and are taken to the nearest hospital, where it is discovered that the pedestrian was sober but that the driver has concentrations of alcohol in his blood that are well above the legal limit. There is only one emergency bed available in the hospital. Moreover, the hospital is a private one; the driver has medical insurance, but the pedestrian has none' (Le Grand, 1991).

He asks the following questions:

'In this situation, who should receive priority treatment? Should it be the pedestrian, on the grounds that she was not at fault? Or should it be the driver, who has the means to pay for the treatment? ... On the assumption that both are equally injured, who should get the emergency bed? Since it is impossible to treat both, the only way of achieving "equal" treatment for equal need is for neither to get treated: a ludicrous outcome. A less strict interpretation of the principle might require allocating the bed on the toss of a coin: each then has an equal probability of obtaining treatment. Yet this seems rather arbitrary: would we really be content if the coin landed in such a way that the drunken driver was treated while the pedestrian died from her injuries?'(Le Grand, 1991).

He gives as an answer the response:

'I think most people would find it more acceptable to allocate the bed to the pedestrian, on the grounds that the driver was, to a large extent, at fault for his predicament, whereas she was not' (Le Grand, 1991).

Preliminary Comment

As shall become clear, there are more ethical questions raised by Le Grand's example than there might appear to be. For instance, there is an ambiguity in Le Grand's formulation of the matter. Who should receive priority treatment? This is not necessarily the same question as: to whom should one allocate the treatment? It is not clear which of these questions Le Grand imagines he is addressing: he seems to oscillate between them.

To say that, were it to occur, such and such would be the morally preferable outcome is not the same thing as saying that what some specified person ought to do is to make the particular decision which brings such and such about. There can be a relevant difference between that which happens and that which is done. It might very well be for the best if, say, great-aunt Freda were to pass away even although no one has a duty to kill her: we all might have a duty not to kill her and some people might have the added duty of trying to ensure that she is not killed.

It might be best, especially if he were to be fairly convicted, that a particular accused and guilty person were declared by a jury to be guilty of a particular crime. One might be pretty sure or even 'know' that the person is guilty and yet applaud the members of a jury – who might well agree with one that the accused, indeed, 'did it' – for returning a not guilty verdict on the grounds that their duty was to consider solely the evidence presented and decide whether, beyond reasonable doubt, it proved the prosecution's case. What might be thought of as 'cosmic justice' and 'panoramic fairness' are often thwarted by honest citizens performing their mundane duties.

Le Grand claims that it would be a ludicrous outcome if neither of the potential patients is treated. This may be so. However, it is not a ludicrous point of view that there are some sorts of decisions that people ought not to make no matter what are the consequences of the failure to make them. Sometimes, when people perform their duties and do, in particular circumstances what they ought to do – and this might be to refuse to make a particular sort of decision – the outcome can seem to be ludicrous. Yet, to do their duty in such circumstances is, perhaps, what people ought to do.

For instance, consider the situation, discussed by Tong, in the early days of *in vitro* fertilisation when surplus embryos were created. What should be done with them? As Tong writes:

'Although modified-protectionists and non-protectionists saw nothing immoral in a couple's requests that their surplus embryos be discarded, full-protectionists [as Tong calls those who consider that an embryo at any stage of development is morally equivalent to a normal human being] claimed that such discards constituted ex utero abortions. They insisted that women should accept all the embryos into their wombs rather than throw any of them away: Better to risk a multiple birth than to deprive any one child of life' (Tong, 1997).

Some of them thought that that is what ought to be done even when the predictable outcome was the 'ludicrous' one that all of the resultant fetuses, because there were so many of them, would die. One might not agree with this position but it is not readily dismissible as 'ludicrous'.

Similarly, when some decisions can or must be made and resultant actions can or must be performed, often there are some reasons which should not be allowed to determine them even when these reasons can lead to the same outcomes as would other reasons including good ones. In this regard, Le Grand dismisses in too cursory a manner the procedure of coin tossing and its metaphorical equivalents. Often, it matters not merely what is done but why what is done is done. A reason which is neither good nor bad can be better than a bad reason for a decision even when the decision is, in both cases, the same. In any case, there is a clear distinction between justifying a procedure and justifying each outcome which a procedure might produce. The jury system, for instance, sometimes produces unfortunate and even 'ludicrous' outcomes. This does not invalidate the procedure. So too it is with coin tossing.

For instance, suppose that it fell to the lot of the captain of a sinking ship to decide what ten passengers were to be allocated to the ten available places in the doomed and heavily populated ship's only life raft. In terms of the outcome of the decision, we might suppose, as might the captain, that it does not matter which particular ten people are chosen. Suppose that there are ten and only ten white passengers aboard. Some people might think that it would be better, independently of the outcome of the decision, to choose ten people on a systematically random basis rather than to choose them on the basis of their colour even if, by remarkable chance, the random system happened to allocate the ten places to the same ten white people. *Why* things are done and not merely *what* is done can matter and in the absence of a good reason for making a decision, a reason which is not a bad one can suffice.

Le Grand's example is a fascinating one. From the host of questions which it might raise, we shall address the following (possibly overlapping) two. To whom would it be better that the treatment were given and why would it be better? If someone other than the potential patients makes the decision as to who will be treated, who should the person choose and why should the person choose him or her? It matters, as we shall see, who makes this choice.

Is the fundamental moral consideration, as Le Grand suggests, 'that the driver was, to a large extent, at fault for his predicament whereas she was not'? No, we shall suggest, it is not. Even in relation to the question of what should happen in this situation this is not precisely the central nor is it the only consideration. In relation to the question of what decisions specific allocators should make, it should not be a consideration at all.

What, Were it to Happen, Would be Best?

Who should get the treatment: the driver or the pedestrian? What should happen? On what basis or bases might a moral commentator, who is *hors de combat* and not an agent in the situation at issue, prefer it to turn out that one rather than the other of the injured people is given treatment (Smith, 1976)? If everything possibly pertinent could be taken into account, for instance, but not merely, a calculus of all the possible consequences of treating one rather than the other of the injured people and, for instance, a consideration of 'fairness' and 'justice' for all those affected directly and indirectly by the case, what would correctly be adjudged the best thing to happen?

The question would seem to be unanswerable. Certainly, the situation, as presented by Le Grand, is not sufficiently specified to warrant a confidently presented conclusion. Perhaps the correct answer might be that there is no morally preferable outcome other than, perhaps, that it is better that one rather than none of them is treated. Perhaps the claims of both people to treatment are in moral equipoise. These two people are not the only morally relevant ones in the entire picture and nor are their claims the only morally relevant ones. Perhaps in equipoise are the overall moral case for favouring the treatment of the pedestrian and the overall moral case for favouring the treating of the driver.

It might turn out that the driver of the car has numerous dependent children and numerous friends who would be made very unhappy by his death while the pedestrian is a misanthrope who would be missed and grieved for by no one.

What if, overall, the man is morally a far better person than the woman? Perhaps this is the first time that he has ever driven a car when drunk; perhaps he was, stupidly but not maliciously, on his way to the chemist with an urgent prescription for a sick child. Perhaps the now sober pedestrian frequently drives a car when she is intoxicated and perhaps, drunk or sober, she abuses her children.

Taking a broad view, the ages, general health and life expectancy of the driver and pedestrian might well enter into the picture. What if the driver is nineteen years old and the pedestrian is ninety one?

What would be the consequences of treating one rather than the other? If the pedestrian is treated rather than the driver, that might tend towards the discouragement of people to take out private medical insurance and, overall, that might be a good or it might be a bad thing. Would the treating of the pedestrian rather than the driver discourage people from drunk driving? It might or it might not.

A case can be made for saying that it would be better if it happened that the driver were treated. A case can be made for saying that it would be better if it happened that the pedestrian were treated.

Consider, first of all, the case for preferring the treatment of the driver. How did it come about that the private hospital was available for the possible treatment of these injured people? Suppose that, were it not for the driver and others who, like him, took out health insurance both the driver and pedestrian would have perished for want of a sufficiently handy hospital. Looked at in this way, it might seem unfair if the woman, who did not help to provide for the presence of the hospital were treated rather than the man who did.

When the man purchased his health insurance, was there a specification that treatment would be withheld were he to be drunk when he required it or, say, injured as the result of an accident caused while he was drunk in charge of a vehicle? If there was, then the man, no less than the woman is without health insurance cover for the period which is being considered. If there was not, then, perhaps it would be unfair were he not to be treated rather than the pedestrian. If, on the grounds of his drunkenness, he were to be denied treatment then this would be as if he were robbed – precisely when he needs it – of what he reasonably thought he had purchased.

It would seem odd, to say the least, to argue that the driver's health insurance should not count in favour of his preferential treatment. Suppose that two other identical accidents were to occur at the same time as this one and that in one of them, the drunk driver has private health insurance while the pedestrian has none and that in the other, the pedestrian has private health insurance while the driver has none. Suppose that both pedestrians are taken to a private hospital (B) which has only one emergency bed available and that both drunk drivers are taken to a private hospital (C) which has only one emergency bed available. In hospital B, who should get the treatment?; the pedestrian with the insurance or the pedestrian without it? The pedestrian with it, surely! It would be very odd to deny that in hospital C, the driver with private insurance has, *ceteris paribus,* the stronger claim to be given priority treatment and that it would be better were he given it. Similarly, it would be curious to say that the drunk driver's possession of health insurance should count for nothing, even if it should not be decisive, in what we might call hospital A of Le Grand's original example. (Notice how, as Le Grand specifies the situation, it is difficult readily to compare like with like.)

Suppose, by the way, that the sober pedestrian and the drunk driver had arrived not at a private hospital but at hospital D – an NHS or other state funded one. Might there still be a case for preferring it to happen that the insured driver is treated? We are not sure. There might be. Perhaps it depends upon the context in which the insurance and lack of insurance occurs and the reasons why the driver is insured and the pedestrian is not. Perhaps the driver is insured because he is an industrious, thoughtful and thrifty sort of person while the pedestrian is a feckless, lazy spendthrift who sometimes thought about acquiring health insurance but, while she was in funds, never quite got round to getting it. If someone must perish in this situation, perhaps, other things being equal, it would be less bad were it to be the feckless and lazy person, if such the pedestrian were to be.

But, of course, other things, we know, are not equal and this is the basis for preferring it to happen that the pedestrian were treated. The driver was drunk and when drunk, he injured both the pedestrian and himself. Not only, as Le Grand stresses, was he at fault for his own injuries while she was not at fault for hers: he was at fault for her injuries as well. It would seem most unfair in the circumstances were he to be treated for his injuries rather than she for hers. One might think: it is bad enough for him to have caused the injury to the woman in the first place but intolerable that he should then doubly wound her, as it were, by being the cause of her failure to receive treatment. One might say that it would be poetic justice in the circumstances were she rather than he to receive the required treatment. He more than she was the author of the accident: it is fitting that he rather than she should bear the bad consequences.

There might too be a case for saying that, even if the driver had been sober, and not morally or legally at fault, it would still be fairer if the woman rather than the man were treated because of his relative authorship of the accident. When the man drove his car, he voluntarily ran the risk of producing and suffering from the sort of accident which subsequently occurred. When the pedestrian was injured, it was not as the consequence, since she was on the pavement, of the sort of accident which pedestrians by their behaviour run the risk of causing.

What if the accident were caused by the sudden illness of the driver where, although the driver was drunk at the time, the illness was unrelated to the drunkenness and would have resulted in the accident even if the driver had been sober? In this case, the accident was not the fault of the driver (although the driver was – irrelevantly? – at fault in being drunk while driving a car just as the woman might have been – irrelevantly? – at fault in being in charge of a dog which, let us say, she allowed to foul the pavement and, say, in having in her possession, for an intended unlawful use, an offensive weapon). It is not clear what one should say about a situation such as this. Perhaps even if the driver was sober when such an illness overtook him it would be fairer were the pedestrian to be treated on the grounds, again, that he voluntarily entered into – but she did not – a course of action which can produce the sort of accident which ensued.

The driver in this situation, since he is drunk, is in breach of his moral and legal duties. One might feel that it is fitting that he is punished in some way. However, it is worth suggesting that whether or not the man deserves punishment might well be unrelated to the question of whether it would be better were the pedestrian rather than he to receive the only available hospital treatment no matter how much Le Grand's example seems to force the two issues together. In any case, the driver has not been tried for drunk driving, far less found guilty of having committed it: his side of the story remains to be told.

Not only is the driver in breach of his moral and legal duties but he has infringed the moral and legal rights of the pedestrian who, it would seem, has a moral and legal right not to be hit, while she is on the pavement, by a motor car driven by someone who is drunk. It would seem to be fitting that the driver compensates her in some way. Again, it is perhaps a mistake to fuse the issue of compensation with that of priority hospital treatment. However, if the pedestrian does not receive the treatment, it would appear that compensation would not be possible in any other way.

The situation might be different if the injuries were of a different sort. Suppose, say, that both received injuries to their fingers and that if treatment were not given immediately, their fingers would be deformed. If only one of them could be treated and if the drunk driver were a concert pianist, it might be better if he were treated rather than the non-musical pedestrian and if, subsequently, he paid her a large sum of money in compensation for her injuries and deformity.

The best thing to happen in Le Grand's example, some people might think, would be for the driver, somehow, to be aware of the situation and of what he had done and to say that the pedestrian rather than he should be treated. If the motorist were voluntarily to transfer his health insurance rights to the pedestrian, then it might be thought that, in the circumstances, this would be the most desirable thing to happen. However, such a transfer is not possible with standard health insurance schemes. (If it were, healthy people would be paid by rich, unhealthy people to takeout health insurance policies with a view to their subsequent transfer.) Perhaps the best thing to happen would be for the driver to forfeit his own treatment and, in addition, pay the hospital for the treatment of the pedestrian.

What Ought to be Done?

Who should get the treatment: the driver or the pedestrian? What ought to be done? Why ought what ought to be done be done? To whom should a provider of treatment allocate the treatment? On what basis or bases might a decision maker who is an active agent in the situation choose properly to discriminate between the injured people when allocating treatment?

I

Consider, first of all, a slight modification of Le Grand's example. Suppose that the injured people were taken not to a private hospital but to the private house of an unemployed doctor who had in his house, let us imagine, the necessary facilities to perform an emergency operation on one but only on one of the people. Who should he choose to treat? It is not at all obvious what the doctor should do or what should be his reasons for doing it.

Ought the doctor to do anything? Suppose he realised that his favourite television programme was about to start and that, in order to watch it, he decided to treat neither of them. This would be uncharitable behaviour and, on that basis, morally condemnable but he would not necessarily be acting in a way which was an infringement of the rights of the potential patients. Does either of them have a right against the doctor that he gives him or her treatment? It is not obvious that either does.

Perhaps the doctor should decide that he should give treatment to one of them if only one of them can be given treatment. However, it does not follow from that that he should make a reflective decision about which of the two people should receive the treatment. Apart from anything else, time taken to make a decision is time which will not be available to give treatment in. If he takes time to decide who he ought to treat, there might well be no-one left alive to treat.

To toss a coin, if there is one to hand, might be a good procedure for the doctor to adopt. It has the merit of speediness. (It is not clear that equality or equal probability of treatment is an important consideration in this instance.) In addition, it might spare the doctor from the psychological torment both at the time and thereafter of having to make and of having made an horrendously stressful and unreasonably difficult decision.

Perhaps one should not think that the doctor in this situation has a moral problem to solve or a moral question to answer if 'problem' suggests 'solution' and 'question' suggests 'correct answer'. What he is faced with, rather, is a dilemma. How best can he cope with it? The doctor did not invite upon himself this predicament. How he can survive it tolerably is itself an important element of the situation. To a large extent, it is the doctor's own business what he decides to do. Various people might, as Le Grand suggests, prefer it to turn out that the pedestrian rather than the driver is treated but the doctor is not answerable to them.

Must the doctor consider the decision of who to treat as, fundamentally, an ethical one? After all when, say, a baker sells bread and a butcher meat, they do not and need not regard every transaction as one necessitating ethical deliberation. The first to come who is willing and able to pay for the bread and the meat receives it. The unemployed doctor, like the rest of us requires money to live the sort of life which he desires and to provide his family and himself with, for instance, food and health care. Suppose that he were to treat the insured driver rather than the uninsured pedestrian on the grounds that he is more likely to be paid for his treatment of him. It is not obvious, to say the least, that such a decision for such a reason would be morally wrong or deserving of blame or censure.

We are dealing with a situation, as implied by Le Grand, where the driver knew that he was drunk, had no good reason for driving whilst drunk, the accident was caused by his inebriated state and the pedestrian was blameless. However, we make here the rather obvious observation that none of this follows simply from the fact that the driver had an illegal level of alcohol in his blood when he arrived at the hospital. After all, in the film *North by Northwest,* the character played by James Mason forces the character played by Cary Grant first to drink a bottle of bourbon and then to drive a car down the twisting coast road. An accident occurs, followed by over two hours of mayhem. But the whole premise of the film is that none of this is the fault of the character played by Cary Grant, a judgement with which we feel Le Grand would concur.

What can the doctor reasonably be assumed to *know* in this situation? Suppose that he knows that the man is drunk, that he was driving the car and that the pedestrian was sober and on the pavement walking her dog at the time of the accident. He knows too, somehow, let us suppose, that the driver has private health insurance whilst the pedestrian has none. He cannot know, however, which of the two is, morally, the better person. He cannot know which of them, overall, is more deserving of the treatment. He cannot know what, overall, will be the consequences of treating one of them rather than the other.

Suppose that the doctor made the decision to favour the person with health insurance. He might imagine, say, that the presence of the insurance was an indication, however reliable, of comparative wealth. He might take the view that, other things being equal and given that he could not save both of them, it would be better to save the person who seemed to be richer. Could his action be considered morally wrong if he were to proceed on that basis? Surely not. What moral principle would such a decision breach?

The doctor might take the view that the taking out of health insurance is a possible sign of foresight, initiative and self-reliance. He might feel that he ought, accordingly to treat the driver. Again, it is not obvious that it would be reasonable to condemn the decision of the doctor however much one might prefer to see the survival of the sober pedestrian and no matter that, were one to have been the doctor, one might have chosen differently.

In general, people with private health insurance are healthier than those without it. This is because of the so-called 'adverse selection' problem: health insurance companies screen potential policy holders; people who are seriously ill or who have a likelihood of becoming seriously ill will have difficulty in getting private health insurance cover. The doctor might favour the treatment of the insured driver on the grounds that the successful treatment of him is likely to result in the saving of a longer and healthier life than the successful treatment of the uninsured person. A similar sort of argument is used at present in the NHS to favour the treatment of younger rather than older patients. That such an action for such a reason would be wrong is not at all obvious.

Consider the situation where, unlike the doctor and the driver, the female pedestrian is black. Suppose that the doctor treated the pedestrian rather than the driver because he was afraid of being unfairly attacked for being a racist and/or a sexist. Would it be wrong to do this for that reason? Would it be moral cowardice? Would it be, even if not morally laudable, excusable?

II

Consider now the instance, as in Le Grand's formulation, where both driver and pedestrian are taken to a private hospital. Imagine that a specified hospital administrator has the job of deciding which of them will be treated. Here, unlike in the case of the unemployed doctor, the medical resources concerned do not belong to the administrator: he has responsibilities towards his employers regarding the allocation of these resources; he has too, even if indirectly, duties towards the insured driver which the unemployed doctor did not have and duties which he, the administrator, does not have towards the uninsured person.

The private hospital will not normally proceed on the basis of treating patients for nothing in preference to patients who will pay. One might assume that, in his capacity as an employee of the hospital, the administrator is obliged to disregard the fact that the driver was drunk while in charge of a motor vehicle unless there is some specified clause in his contract which obliges him to take this into account. Similarly, one might assume that the administrator is obliged as an employee of the hospital to give treatment to, in this instance, preferential treatment to the insured driver.

What the administrator ought to do *qua* employee would seem to be clear-cut. Of course, there are circumstances where human beings have obligations *qua* human beings which can over-ride such role-based obligations even when the roles are voluntarily adopted. 'I was only following orders' will not always be an adequate defence of our actions. By the same token neither will be the claim: 'I was trying to further what I consider to be a more important end than that which I had previously agreed to further'. Perhaps, what the human being who is the administrator ought to do in the circumstances is to allocate treatment for the driver rather than the pedestrian. That he would have a higher moral obligation of some sort to act otherwise is possible but not manifest.

III

What if both injured people had arrived not at a private hospital but at an NHS or other state-funded one? Imagine that an administrator who was directly or indirectly an employee of the state had the responsibility of deciding who of the two were to be treated. What ought he to do and on what grounds?

It is not the job or business of such employees to mete out punishments for the breaches of legal or moral rules. Such an administrator might think, say, that it would be better if the sober pedestrian rather than the drunk driver were treated on the grounds, for instance, that the driver but not the pedestrian was a fault. However, it is not the job of such a person to make decisions on the basis of what he or she thinks would, overall, be productive of a morally apt outcome.

It is easier to say what such a person should *not* do and should *not* take into account than to say what he or she should do and why he or she should do it. The drunkenness of the driver, if it is not medically relevant to the likely effectiveness of treatment should be ignored by the administrator unless there is some legitimate, properly established rule which says otherwise. Similarly, the administrator should ignore the possession by the driver of medical insurance (unless Parliament has passed legislation which indicates that he should not).

Andersson makes the interesting and plausible claim that:

'A community can make demands on its members that it cannot make on foreigners; but foreigners then do not have an equal right to be cared for by the community' (Andersson, 1995). Making the simplifying assumption that both injured people are citizens of the state in question, one can say that the administrator, as an official or quasi-official and representative of the state has a duty – which the unemployed doctor does not have and the administrator of a private hospital does not have in the same way – to consider the claims to treatment of both people impartially and that both people have corresponding rights to have their claims -implicit although they would be in the circumstances – considered impartially. In what would impartial treatment consist in the circumstances? It is not clear. To toss a coin might be an appropriate response to the requirement of impartiality. The administrator here, like, say, a judge, a member of a jury or the marker of a student's examination script is morally obliged to deal with the case solely in terms of particular relevant criteria: various considerations such as, say, plausible speculation about the moral worth of the injured people, which it would be permissible or even morally obligatory for the unemployed doctor, as a private individual human being, to take into account are out of bounds to him or her in his or her official capacity.

Obviously, such hospital administrators are not expected to be mere automatons automatically applying bureaucratic rules. They are required to use their judgement but they are required to use their professional judgement in defined spheres: theirs is not the task of deciding what, morally, ought to happen nor what, overall, would be morally preferable outcomes of decisions to treat or not to treat particular potential patients.

Private Health Care

It might be thought that Le Grand's example tells against private health insurance. It is unfair, some people might argue, that people should be able to pay for preferential health care and use their money to 'jump the queue'. If it turns out that the insured driver rather than the un-insured pedestrian is treated when the administrator in the private hospital does his job properly, then this, some people would argue, is a reason for disfavouring, and making illegal, perhaps, private health insurance and private medicine. Health care, because of the effect it can have on whether people live or die, should not, some people might say, be available for sale.

We see the situation differently. It is not that, somehow, the driver's possession of private health insurance deprived the pedestrian of treatment if the driver rather than she were treated in the private hospital. If there were no private hospital there, neither would have been treated. If both injured people had turned up at the private hospital and neither of them had private insurance, it does not follow that the pedestrian rather than the driver would have been or should have been treated.

One might concoct an example similar to Le Grand's but concerning food rather than health care. For instance, suppose that two people – a child-abusing, murderous woman and a sensitive, caring, law-abiding man – have an aeroplane accident in remote mountains which is totally the fault of the woman pilot, who was flying in a drug-induced haze. They arrive, let us imagine, several days latter, near starvation, at a local market where there is food enough only to secure the survival of one of them. The woman has sufficient money to purchase the food. The man has no money at all.

The conventional market outcome would be for the woman, who has the money, to be given preferential treatment and, in return for the money, given the food. It might well be that, morally, the better outcome would be for the man rather the woman to receive the food necessary for survival. If neither of them had money, then there might be the 'ludicrous' outcome that neither of them was given food and both of them starved to death. However, this particular example does not prove nor even suggest that, as a general arrangement, food should not be available for sale on a commercial basis.

In general, the market, subject to possible regulation, is the most appropriate way to produce and allocate food even although food is necessary for human survival (McLachlan, 1998). In times of food scarcity, the market mechanism is often restricted or replaced by a quantity-rationing system. During the Second World War, general food shortages in the U.K. led to the adoption of an official rationing system. Subsequently, in periods of specific shortages of particular foods, such as sugar, shops impose an unofficial rationing procedure by setting a ceiling to the amount any one consumer can purchase.

These are regarded as exceptional responses to unusual circumstances. When normal conditions of supply return, the market is re-instated; there is no general desire for rationing to be retained for longer than is necessary.

Whilst many families would wish to eat more and better, there is no general perception of a food shortage in the present U.K. economy. However, there is thought to be a shortage of health provision – fuelled, the expectation, that is, by the existence of queues for NHS treatment. Le Grand's example gains credibility, perhaps, from such a perception. However, it is wrong to say that such a shortage is the result of private health provision (as it would be wrong to blame a shortage of books in public libraries on the existence and success of private bookshops such as Waterstone's and Dillon's). It is, rather, the result of the failure of the electorate to vote into power a party committed to substantially increasing the level of resources going into health care.

Conclusion

The example of the drunk driver and the sober pedestrian given by Le Grand is a fascinating one. The issues raised are more complex and less clear-cut, perhaps, than they first appear. In particular, the questions of what would be better to happen were it to happen and of what people ought to do in the situation are worth separating. The moral situation of an administrator in a private hospital should be distinguished from that of a private individual as well as, possibly, from that of an NHS or other state-employed official. Despite what Le Grand might be thought to imply, it is not the case that, unequivocally, the drunkenness of the driver establishes that the pedestrian rather than he should be treated or that, unequivocally, the driver's possession of health insurance is morally irrelevant.

Recall, if you will, Le Grand's initial example of the insured drunk driver and the sober uninsured pedestrian and his question:

'In this situation, who should receive priority treatment? Should it be the pedestrian, on the grounds that she was not at fault? Or should it be the driver, who has the means to pay for the treatment?' (Le Grand, 1991).

If the question is considered in global moral terms regarding what decision about priority treatment, overall, would be better, the question would seem to be unanswerable. Perhaps the correct answer, whether or not it could be knowable as such, is that there is, overall, no moral preference for the treatment of one rather than the other. Perhaps, too, one or other of them should receive the priority treatment but on grounds other than that suggested by Le Grand. Again, if the question is considered to be about what an active private moral agent in the situation ought to do and for what reasons, no one definitive answer readily emerges.

If the question were about what an administrator in an NHS (or other state-funded) hospital ought to do were both injured people to have been delivered there, then, again the correct answer is not obvious. It seems clear enough that the administrator should ignore *both* the drunkenness *and* the possession or non-possession of health insurance. Other than that, nothing much, with justified confidence, can be said. Perhaps to toss a coin or, metaphorically, to do something of that sort would be the best procedure to follow. It would be beside the point to say that this procedure might produce a result which some people might not like. For instance, juries sometimes in particular cases reach the 'wrong' verdict; that is not an argument against the system of trials by jury as an appropriate procedure for deciding some particular issues.

If the question is about what an administrator in a private hospital ought to decide to do in that capacity then the answer is clear enough. The administrator should decide that the driver is treated although not perhaps, as in Le Grand's formulation because he 'has the means to pay for the treatment' – the issue does not revolve around the *means* that people have or have not – but because *he already has paid* for his health insurance.

Are there any policy implications which could be drawn from Le Grand's example? There might be but it is not clear whether or not there are. As has been argued very convincingly by, for instance, Brazier, hard cases can make bad laws (Brazier, 1997).

One might argue that there are certain risks – such as some of the risks of being injured while drunk-driving (and performing certain other illegal actions) – which one should not be allowed to insure one's self against. Perhaps a good case could be made on this basis. Yet, it is not clear that the operation of such a rule – somehow specified – would be applicable in the situation envisaged by Le Grand. In all likelihood, what would happen under the operation of such a rule is that the driver would be treated in the private hospital and then, after due process when and if his legal guilt were to be established, he would be required to pay the hospital for the treatment which they gave him on the assumption, which proved to be false, that his insurance covered that treatment. The rule could hardly be that the insurance of privately insured patients does not hold while they happen to be drunk. The administrator in the private hospital, we would suggest, would be required to act on the assumption that the insurance of the driver was in order. The administrator can hardly be expected in the circumstances of the emergency, and without the driver having an opportunity to present a defence, to act as judge, jury and, in effect, executioner.

If, when people perform the duties of their employment in private and in state funded hospitals, the outcome concerning priority treatment in emergency cases is considered to be undesirable, consideration could be given to changing the laws, rules and expectations within which these people work, thereby changing their duties of employment.

Should the rules under which the NHS operates be changed to ensure that in a situation such as that described by Le Grand, an administrator, acting upon them, would give priority to the sober pedestrian rather than to the drunk driver? We do not think so. People who commit crimes such as drunk-driving should be punished but they should be punished by the courts after having been given a fair trial and not, in the absence of one, by hospital administrators.

It were to be decided that, say, the moral worth, social usefulness and/or criminality of citizens should be a relevant consideration in the allocation of NHS treatment – and the suggestion is a startling one – it is not clear how or that a pertinent rule could be formulated and enforced by NHS administrators. What possible rule could an NHS administrator apply which would be reasonable, just and fair and whose application would result, in the situation outlined by Le Grand, in the pedestrian being given treatment rather than the driver because of the moral and legal culpability of the driver? It is no use saying, for instance, that the driver was responsible for his injury (and hers) while the pedestrian was not responsible for hers since this responsibility is not something which it is possible for any one, in the context of the emergency, to ascertain nor something which it is appropriate for the administrator, in the capacity of an NHS administrator, to make a judgement about – far less such a judgment which is acted upon – in any context.

*By Hugh V. McLachlan and J. Kim Swales, from *Health Care Analysis*, Vol. 7, No.1, pp. 5-21.

References

Andersson, J.O. (1995) 'Real Freedom, Democratic Community and Sustainable Development as Fundamental Values' in Economic Enquiry. In R. Eriksson and M. Jantii (Eds.), *Economic Value and Ways of Life*. Aldershot: Avebury.

Brazier, M. (1997) 'Hard Cases Make Bad Law'. *Journal of Medical Ethics* 23, 341-343.

Le Grand, J. (1991) *Equity and Choice: An Essay in Economics and Applied Philosophy*. London and New York: Harper Collins Academic.

McLachlan, H.V. (1995) Smokers, Virgins, Equity and Health Care Costs. *Journal of Medical Ethics* 21, 209-213.

McLachlan, H.V. (1998) Justice, Rights and Health Care. *International Journal of Sociology and Social Policy* 18(3/4).

Smith, A. (1976) *The Theory of Moral Sentiments* (Edited by D. Raphael and A. Macfie). Oxford: Clarendon Press.

Tong, R. (1997) *Feminist Approaches to Bioethics*. Oxford: Westview Press.

Chapter Eighteen

Scotland, Health and Inequality*

'Health! Health! Health!' Such would seem to be a mantra of the Scottish Executive. However, the suggested *rationale* for its proposed approach to health policy is unconvincing.

According to *Working Together for a Healthier Scotland* (Cm 3583), health policy should be geared towards improving health and reducing health inequalities. In this Scottish Green Paper, it is proposed that the NHS should have as its main aim the improvement in health rather than the treatment of illness. It is said too that: 'Above all, we need to attack the inequalities which scar our health record'. (p. 1-2)

The claims of this Scottish Green Paper are an echo of the Report of the Commission on Social Justice, set up by the late John Smith where it is said that: 'The first issue we address is how best to promote good health and reduce health inequalities'. (See *Social Justice: Strategies for National Renewal*, Vintage, 1994, p.285)

In this paper we wish to make the following arguments. First, the proposal in the Scottish Green Paper represents not just one policy but two. These are: improving health and increasing health equality. Secondly, the pursuit of health equality almost certainly involves a trade-off in terms of lower average health. Finally, the attempt to achieve health equality is likely to be inconsistent with the more fundamental goal of equality of entitlement to health treatment.

Two Policy Aims

A central problem is that the improvement of the general level of health and the reduction of health inequalities is not *one* policy aim. They are, rather, two different policy aims. If there is a conflict between the promotion of health and the reduction of health inequalities which of the two goals should be preferred? On what grounds should it be preferred? Some steps – perhaps most or even all steps – to promote good health might increase health inequalities. For instance, health education schemes, if they have any beneficial effects at all, typically influence different people and different categories of people differently.

Should the Reduction of Health Inequalities be a Policy Aim?

For the sake of the present argument, let us assume (what is debatable) that the promotion of health is a meaningful and reasonable aim for a government or governmental agency to pursue. It is not at all clear that the reduction of health inequalities *per se* is a reasonable or even a meaningful aim of governmental policy. It is not clear why, other than on grounds of social aesthetics or dogmatic egalitarianism, inequalities in health – whether between men and women, rich or poor, black or white or whatever – should in themselves be considered undesirable.

Let us begin by considering a costless change that improves the health of one person, or one particular social group, whilst leaving the health of everyone else unchanged. Should such an improvement be discouraged if it increases health inequality? We believe not. Imagine such a policy measure whose sole effect was an increase in the life expectancy of, say, middle class people, or of white people or of black people or of male, middle class, white people. We would be in favour of implementing any such scheme. Why not?

Infant mortality rates are higher in Scotland in more socially deprived localities. It would certainly be good if the infant mortality rates in the poorest areas of Scotland were to be reduced. What if they were to be reduced and, at the same time, the infant mortality rates of the best-off area were also to be reduced? Would that not be better still, even if health inequalities were not reduced? Why the stress on reducing inequalities?

Imagine the reverse situation: should the health of an individual or group ever be reduced simply to promote health equality? Women in Scotland live, on average, longer than men do. It would be possible to eliminate this inequality. For instance, the S.A.S. could be employed to kill a sufficient number of women such that, on average, the life expectancy of men and women in Scotland became the same. Not only would these means be unacceptable but, we suggest, so too would be the end of such a policy. Again, if the life-styles of the 'working' and 'middle' classes, as conventionally conceived, were to become more similar, then health inequalities might decrease. However, the general level of health might decline in Britain depending on whether or not working or middle class patterns of, for instance, smoking and consuming fresh fruit and vegetables became the norms. Similarly, if, say, the behaviour and circumstances of men and women become more similar, their health might become more equal but, overall, less good. Would the Scottish Executive endorse these changes? In practice it seems not. At present an advertising campaign aimed at reducing smoking by young women is being run in Scotland. On health equality grounds such trends in female smoking, i.e. increasing rates of smoking, should be encouraged, rather than resisted. Equality for the sake of equality seems to us an absurd principle in the context of the average health of different social groups.

What is Wrong with Health Inequality?

Suppose that working class people were not allowed to vote. Suppose, say, that working class people were given longer prison sentences than were middle class people who were equally guilty of having committed the same offences. Such inequalities would, manifestly, be wrong and unjust. However, not all inequalities are unjust; not all inequalities are wrong. If, on average, people who are poor are more likely to suffer from ill health and to die younger than people who are rich, then – whether or not it might be a good idea to try to install laws and public policies to alter the situation – the situation is not necessary an injustice nor the result of one. Those individuals who suffer from ill health and those individuals who die relatively young are not necessarily being deprived of the enjoyment *of a right*.

Who or what has a duty to ensure that these particular individuals do not have an unusually short life span? Who or what has a duty to ensure that these particular individuals are not more unhealthy than richer people tend to be? Who or what has any other related obligation concerning the health and life span of these particular people?

Had we been born in, say, the third rather than the second millennium or in Japan rather than Scotland, or in Scotland but of richer parents, then we might have had a greater chance of better health and a longer life than we have but this is not a matter of justice and rights: it is a matter of luck. As we have noted already, in present day Scotland women live longer than men. Is this fair? Is it unfair? We do not know. (Perhaps it is neither fair nor unfair: neither just nor unjust.) We most certainly do not think that public policy should be geared towards the elimination of this gender and health inequality.

Sometimes, inequalities are wrong because a larger share for some people necessitates a smaller share for others. Health is not like that. The distribution of health is not a 'zero-sum game'.[1] If, say, we own more land now than we did ten years ago, you might think that our increased land-holding must correspond to the deceased land-holding of some other person or agency: there is only so much land available to be parcelled off. If, however, we are healthier now than we were ten years ago, it would be absurd to imagine that our increase in healthiness was at the expense of someone else's corresponding decrease. Indeed, our conspicuous increased healthiness and happiness may have had on some benevolent and sympathetic people the effect of increasing theirs.

Sometimes, even when they are not unjust, social inequalities are undesirable because they are socially divisive and produce disharmony. Sometimes, on grounds other than justice, policies to reduce inequalities might be justifiable. It is not clear that health inequalities come into this category.

In contemporary Scotland, although some other inequalities might be, inequalities of health are not socially divisive. We might covet, say our neighbour's house or, more likely, the houses of people who stay in better neighbourhoods than we do ourselves but we are not in general envious of other people's health. One reason for this might be that while we might buy, steal or, on some other basis, acquire our neighbour's house, we cannot acquire his health: health is non-transferable

Among the various other reasons is that, in general, people do not tend to think of themselves as being members of social categories, which have, for instance, different life expectancies than other social categories. Why should they? Relative death rates are, in any case, not widely known nor highly visible.

Policy Conflict

If the Scottish Executive is to be set clear – or, perhaps more usefully, vague – goals concerning health, why should they not relate to the promotion of good health and the reduction in ill-health no matter whether or not health inequalities are increased or reduced? One beguiling argument that appears to remove the conflict between the two policies is that the most effective way to improve the general health of the country is to improve the health of the worst to the level of the best.[2] However, this argument is both disingenuous and flawed.

The first problem is that readjusting the supply of health-care resources to those who have presently the worst health will almost certainly reduce the situation of those who at present have the best health. To deny this is to suggest that these individuals presently get no benefit from the health care they receive. However, a policy of health-care resource redistribution might still be consistent with optimising the overall health of the country if those with poor health would benefit particularly strongly from additional resources. However, if this is the case, why be concerned about equality as such? Under these conditions maximising the overall health of the country will automatically bring about health equality.

The truth of the matter is that unless individuals have an identical genetic make-up and make identical life-style choices, there is a conflict between health equality and maximising average health. If they are to embrace these two objectives, how does the Scottish Executive envisage operationalising the resulting trade-off?

Equality of Healthcare Entitlement

A counter to the arguments presented already might take the following form. In general it is an advance that the Scottish Executive should set its targets in terms of health outcomes rather than inputs: this encourages efficiency in the use of resources and recognises the role of preventative medicine. Also, it is wrong to make a fetish of consistency: individuals and organisations often have inconsistent objectives and have to trade off one goal against another in a way that is not made fully explicit. We manage to do it and the outcome is acceptable a lot of the time. Finally, whether one likes it or not, individuals have a desire for "fairness" and "equality", though these can be ill defined and elastic concepts in practice.

However, our concern here is the specific goal of equality in health outcomes. We argue above that there is little evidence that people are particularly concerned with inequality of health outcomes as such. However, there is a lot of evidence that people are concerned with inequality of healthcare entitlement, especially healthcare provided by the NHS. But a commitment to equality of health outcomes seems inconsistent with a commitment to healthcare entitlement. In fact it seems to imply discrimination in the provision of healthcare toward those individuals and groups who at present have poor health. This kind of discrimination ruthlessly pursued is potentially socially divisive, potentially illegal and could undermine the NHS itself.

Some have argued that the desire for equality and fairness is genetically programmed in human beings and is derived from the advantages derived by social groups that shared food in the hunter-gatherer stage of human evolution. This sharing was a form of insurance. Whether this argument is true or false, one of the major strengths of the NHS is that it provides such an all-inclusive form of (health) insurance.[3] This cannot be replicated by private insurance because of adverse selection problems: it is not possible to get private insurance if you are seriously ill. However, within this NHS scheme, it would seem reasonable to expect that individuals had equal health care entitlement.[4]

Different racial groups have different genetic and life-style characteristics that make them differentially healthy. Will there be discrimination in their entitlement to health resources through the NHS in Scotland? Is this legal under anti-discriminatory legislation? Different income groups similarly have, on average, different health status. Will there be discrimination in entitlement to public health care by post-code? It is difficult for individuals to know how much they contribute in taxes to public health provision. However, if groups who are likely to be very health conscious anyway find themselves having lower health care entitlements because of their relatively healthy state, they will withdraw support for the NHS. It is difficult to believe that this is what the Scottish Executive is planning.

Conclusion

Often, people and agencies must, in order to act justly, treat other people equally unless there are relevant grounds for treating them unequally. However, although they are required to justify or desist from unequal treatment which they are responsible for meting out, the Scottish Executive is not required to justify or to remove all Scottish social inequalities which happen to occur. Its concern with the distribution of health – something outwith its moral responsibility and, however much it might *affect* it, beyond its control – as opposed, say, to the distribution of aspects of healthcare is puzzling. The Scottish Executive's philosophy of health policy should, we suggest, be further explained or else abandoned.

*By Hugh V. McLachlan and J. Kim Swales, from *Quarterly Economic Commentary, Fraser of Allander Institute*, 2002, Vol. 27, No. 2, pp. 37-40.

Footnotes

(1) Neither is the distribution of wealth, a notion which is a cornerstone of New Labour economic policy.

(2) This is the form of assertion made in the H.M.Treasury's document on spatial differences in productivity.

(3) Of course, there are other arguments for and against the NHS.

(4) In practice, there are many problems with this notion, though as a broad principle it is sound.

(See *The NHS in Scotland: The Legacy of the Past and the Prospect of the Future*, Chris Nottingham (editor), Ashgate, 2000 for a further discussion of this and related issues. See also *Social Justice, Human Rights and Public Policy*, Hugh V McLachlan, Humming Earth, 2005.)

Chapter Nineteen

Human Reproduction and Rights of Action and of Recipience*

Introduction

What Savulescu has said recently about rights in general and about some suggested rights in particular will be discussed.[1] He was talking about claims for compensation in relation to un-predicted and/ or undisclosed congenital deformities in situations where pregnant women were in consultation with their doctors with regard to their pregnancies. He writes: 'What constitutes a right is a complex question. On one interpretation, rights protect interests. This implies that a right not to be born would exist if a child had an interest in not being born'.[2] He goes on to say: 'I don't know if there is a right not to be born. But there is undoubtedly a right to information and a right to make choices about how many children we have, and when we have them and what kind of children we have'.[3] There is, I agree, a right to information. However, I doubt and shall give a reason for doubting whether the other rights which Savulescu mentions exist.

Rights

Pivotal to the issue is what it means to have a 'right'. Savulescu does not specify whether he is talking about moral rights or legal rights: he seems, sometimes, to be talking about the one and, at other times, about the other. I shall try to analyse both.

Let us look first of all at moral rights. There are at least -and, perhaps, only – two types of moral rights: rights of action and rights of recipience.[4]

One has a right of action, for example, to be naked or to lift from the ground a fallen wild strawberry if, when and insofar as one is not under an obligation to refrain from being naked or to refrain from picking up fallen wild strawberries. These rights of action do not in themselves correspond to the obligations of – nor do they impose obligations on – other people. If and when one has these particular rights of action, other people are not thereby obliged, for instance, to try to help us become naked nor to try to help us pick up a fallen wild strawberry (although they might be so obliged on other grounds). Indeed, someone else, with quicker reflexes, out for a walk in the country might have, no less than us, a right of action to pick up a particular fallen wild strawberry and, before our eyes, lift and eat the strawberry without thereby infringing our rights.

Rights of action are the absences of obligations. On the other hand, rights of recipience of a person are rights which correspond to the duties of another person or persons (or agency or agencies). For instance, if one loans someone £5, then one has a right of recipience to £5 from him or her and he or she has a corresponding duty to give us £5. To talk here of our 'right' and his or her 'duty' is to give different perspectives of the same thing.[5, 6, 7]

Notice that while, on this analysis, all moral rights of recipience can be expressed in terms of duties, not all duties are expressible in terms of rights. For instance, we might have a duty to be charitable where no particular person has a right against us to the receipt of our charity. Notice too that moral rights and duties do not arise solely from such voluntary arrangements as making promises. For instance, independently of our wills and not as a consequence of any private transactions into which we have entered, we have a moral duty not to slander other people (including people we have never met and never transacted with) and they have a corresponding moral right not to be slandered by us.

I suspect that, although legislatures and courts might declare anything at all to be 'legal rights', these legal rights can be expressed in terms of the absence of (or immunity from) specified legal obligations or in terms of the specified obligations of specified parties: otherwise, such so-called 'legal rights' could be considered as mere verbiage. They are like unsigned cheques. Whether or not Kant is correct in claiming that 'ought' implies 'can' i.e. that we can be morally obliged to do such and such only if it is possible for us to do so, it is manifest that some persons can be burdened with legal duties which they cannot possibly fulfil. In such circumstances, there can be persons with specified corresponding legal rights. What they have are akin to dud cheques.

Justice, Rights, Interests and Needs

There is a relationship between justice and rights.[8] [9] One acts unjustly when one fails to perform a duty which corresponds to another's right of recipience. One acts justly when one performs such a duty. There are moral rights of recipience and legal rights of recipience. There is moral justice and legal justice.

It seems to me that, although it might perhaps be unjustly taken from us, much of what we have that is most worth having

– including life itself – was not allocated to us as a moral right but fell to our lot as something else. We might need and/or want and/or have an interest in various things such as, for instance, sex without thereby acquiring a moral right to have them – without, that is, it being the case that some person or agency has thereby a moral duty to provide us with them. We might have particular moral rights that we do not want and do not need. Someone desiring to be dead has a right to life (if there is such a human right) whether he wants to have it or not.

Moral rights stem from moral duties. There is no mechanism which ensures that there will be a connection between, on the one hand, what individual X or agency Y has a moral duty to do and, on the other hand, what individual Z wants, needs or has an interest in. Similarly, the wants, needs and interests of Z do not automatically generate duties on the part of X or Y. If I as a layman knew no less than did a doctor facts which were in the interests of his or her patient to know, my duties (my moral and legal ones) would not be the same as the doctor's. Hence, the rights of the patient relative to me would not be the same as the rights of the patient relative to the doctor. This happens even though the patient's interests pertaining to the information – since it is the same information – are the same in both cases. The rights of the patient do not derive from their interests. Their rights – both moral and legal – flow from the duties of others: such duties might, in a straight-forward or in a roundabout way, be related to their interests. They often are, yet sometimes they are not.

Some legal rights protect some of our interests. Nonetheless, the relationship between legal rights and interests is complex and highly variable. One can have legal rights which one does not need or want or have an interest in. For instance, many Roman Catholics in some countries would prefer not to have the legal rights that pertain to abortion. Our legal rights are a product of the decisions of our politicians and our courts. There is no mechanism to ensure that what emerge as our legal rights will be in our interests or that we will want them or need them. Politicians do not always try to burden agents and agencies with duties whose fulfilment will further the interests of all or even some other citizens. Even when they try, they do not always succeed.

We are sometimes accorded legal rights which cannot or will not be fulfilled. Are such rights in our interests? Even when citizens have legal rights of recipience that are honoured, the appearance that such rights are in their interests can be illusory. Politicians, if they were more honest, would tell the electors that they were proposing to burden them with consequent additional duties every time they promised them new legal rights of recipience. When citizens receive benefits, the citizenry usually pays for them one way or another. Whether, overall, the citizenry would be better off with the benefits and consequent burdens than it would be if it had neither is, more often than not, a moot point.

Savulescu notes with approval that Australian courts seem to have ruled that doctors can be deemed legally guilty of negligence if they fail to disclose to patients information that the patients themselves would have considered relevant to their own best interests. This could happen even if, in line with the Bolam standard, a reasonable body of similar medical practitioners might also have done the same thing in similar circumstances.[3] I do not want a legal right in the U.K. to information of this sort. Furthermore, I think that it is unwise to create such a legal right. Overall, we would be better off without it. There are better uses of doctors' time than the provision of such information. Doctors would need to know far more about their patients than it is their duty to find out in order to be able to provide the information.

Phantom Rights and Actual Duties

I think that Savulescu is correct in saying that pregnant women have a right to information. All the other supposed rights indicated by him are, to say the least, dubious. Even if we have such moral rights, we do not undoubtedly have them. We have a right to information from our doctor because he or she has a duty to give it to us. Our right corresponds to his or her duty. The doctor has a duty to give us particular sorts of information not because it is in our interests to have it (which it might or might not be) but because he or she is a doctor and we are his or her patients. By agreeing to be our doctor and accepting payment for being one, our doctor is morally (and legally) obliged to do certain things. Giving patients relevant information is one of them. We can talk about the rights of the patient to information because we can pin down agents and agencies – doctors, hospitals and health services – who do and can have the corresponding duties. In the other cases, no agent nor agency can reasonably or obviously be said to bear the duties that would correspond to the so-called 'rights' in question.

Consider, for instance, the suggested right to choose how many children to have. Suppose that woman X chooses to have ten children and that she has ten children. Suppose that woman Y chooses to have three children but, in the event, she has no children at all. Suppose that woman Z chooses to have two and she has ten children. In what senses, if any, did X, Y and Z have a right to make the choices they did? Notice that there is a difference between having a right to choose to have a particular number of children (if there is such a right) and a right to have that particular number of children. They have a legal right of action to choose to have as many children as they chose to have and a legal right of action to have as many children as they choose to have (and/or as they have) since they are not legally obliged to refrain from having nor from choosing to have any particular number of children.

It is not clear what if anything can be said about their supposed moral rights of action concerning how many children they have or choose to have. For instance, one of them might have some particular genetically transferable condition which might (but might not) oblige her to desist from having children or, at least, from having many. For other women, becoming pregnant might be and predictably be fatal. A moral duty of self preservation in addition to other duties, including some she has voluntarily incurred, would tend towards obliging her to remain childless.

Even if no person nor agency has the 'moral right' to choose for a woman how many children she has, it does not follow that she must have – by default as it were – such a 'moral right' herself. After all, if a man of modest financial means chooses to have, with a variety of women, five hundred children in order to impress his friends with his virility, most people would say – and it seems true to say – that although he had a legal right of action to make and to try to realise this choice, he had no such moral right. He ought not to have made this choice. He ought not to have had so many children. Similarly, in the economic circumstances she was in, perhaps X should have limited her choice and her children to maybe two, even if this moral obligation did not correspond to the right of any one or thing.

If the number of children that women have does not coincide with the number of children that they chose to have, are they deprived thereby of the fulfilment of a right of recipience? No, they are not. I am sorry for Y, who has no children. I hope that she is given help in order to enable her to have children. However, like all other people, Y has no legal right of recipience to have children. No persons or agencies are failing thereby in their duties if Y remains childless. One might similarly be sorry for people without spouses or 'partners'.

However, no one has a legal right of recipience to be married or to have a partner since no one has the legal duty to marry or to be the partner of any particular person. No person or agency has a legal duty to impregnate Y or to see to it that she is impregnated.

Y, like all other people, does not have a moral right of recipience to have children. No one has a moral duty to ensure that she is impregnated or, that if she is impregnated, the pregnancy runs its course. She might be unattractive and/or infertile. She might be fertile and attractive and yet fail to attract a partner who is acceptable to her. Some people, although not all, would suggest that the woman's husband, if she has one, has a moral duty to try to impregnate her if that is her wish. Even if he has such an obligation to try, he is not obliged to succeed. He might be impotent. She might be sterile. They might be potent and fertile and yet unsuccessful – unlucky – in their attempts to succeed.

I don't know why Z had more children than she chose to have. Perhaps it was due to the absence of totally reliable and risk-free contraception. I think it is a good thing that reliable and reasonably safe contraception exists and I think that it is good that it is made easily and cheaply available. However, it does not follow that it is the duty of the state or of some other agency or person to produce such contraception for Z. It is not the legal duty of any person nor agency to ensure that Z has only two children if two children is what she chooses to have.

Z might have more children than she chose to have because the particular application of the method of contraception she was using was very defective. She might have a legal right to compensation of some sort but she might not. We have, in some circumstances, a legal right not to be misinformed: that is not the same thing as having a legal right to such information that is in our interests to have. It is not the same thing as having a legal right to be fully informed. Even if she has a right to compensation and/or is awarded some, this is not the same thing as having a legal or moral right to choose how many children to have. Apart from anything else, one might have more children than one chose to have for reasons other than this. For instance, one might use a non-defective form of contraception wrongly. A legal right to the provision, if they are marketed, of goods and services of a marketable standard is not the same thing as a right to the number of children that one chooses.

Conclusion

Rights are not, somehow, conjured into reality by the mere desirability of their existence. The terms: 'It would be morally good were Y to have X' and 'Y has a moral right to X' are not synonymous. Moral rights should, I suggest, always be thought of in relationship to duties. Contrary to what Savulescu says it is not manifest or in any way clear-cut that we have "... a right to make choices about how many children we have, and when we have them and what kind of children we have'.[3] It is doubtful whether we have moral rights of recipience to such things. Who or what are the bearers of the corresponding duties? It is far from clear what, if anything, can truly be said in general about the moral rights of action concerning these issues. We have, I believe, and should have legal rights of action to make the sorts of choices mentioned by Savulescu but we do not have nor should we have legal rights of recipience in relation to such choices.

*By Hugh V McLachlan from *Human Reproduction and Genetic Ethics*, 2004, Vol.10, No.2. pp. *45-48*. With kind permission of Springer Sciences and Business Media.

References

(1) Savulescu J., 2002. 'Is there a "right not to be born"?: Reproductive decision making, options and the right to information', *Journal of Medical Ethics*, Vol.28, pp. 65-67.

(2) Savulescu J.. 2002, 'Is there a "right not to be born"?: Reproductive decision making, options and the right to information'. *Journal of Medical Ethics,* Vol.28, p.65.

(3) Savulescu J., 2002, 'Is there a "right not to be born"?: Reproductive decision making, options and the right to information'. *Journal of Medical Ethics*, Vol.28, p.66.

(4) Raphael D.D., 1971, *Problems of political philosophy*, London: Macmillan, p.68.

(5) McLachlan H.V., 1973, 'The right to work'. *Contemporary Review, Vol.* 222, pp.307-311.

(6) McLachlan H.V.,1997. 'Bodies, rights and abortion'. *Journal of Medical Ethics*, Vol.23,pp. 176-180.

(7) O'Neill O.,2002, *Autonomy and Trust in Bioethics*, Cambridge: Cambridge University Press, pp.78-82.

(8) McLachlan H.V.,1998, 'Justice, rights and health care:

A discussion of the report of the Commission on Social Justice' *International Journal of Sociology and Social Policy*, Vol.37, pp.65-84.

(9) McLachlan H.V., 2002, 'Tobacco, taxation and fairness', *Journal of Medical Ethics*, Vol.28, pp.381-383.

Chapter Twenty

Smokers, Virgins, Equity and Health Care Costs*

Abstract

Julian Le Grand's case for saying that it would be equitable if smokers and smokers alone were to pay the costs of smoking-related health care is considered and found to be deficient.

Should smokers (and smokers alone) pay the costs of smoking-related health care? No – I shall suggest – at least in contemporary Britain, they should not. I will consider the question with specific reference to the philosophy of public health finance of Le Grand. This philosophy of Le Grand's is based upon a very dubious notion of 'equity'. Nonetheless, what he says about smoking and health care costs is of interest in its own right and might well be attractive to some people who have no knowledge of or interest in his views about 'equity'.

According to Le Grand: 'Situations where one person is disadvantaged relative to another due to factors beyond either's control are commonly judged inequitable; situations where the disadvantage arises because of differences in individual choices freely made are not. Equity depends on the extent of individual choice' [1]. I do not think that people normally conceive of equity and inequity in this way. More importantly, they should not conceive of equity and inequity after this particular fashion. I shall use the term 'equity' in what I think is the normal usage, whereby, 'equity', 'fairness' and 'justice' are identical or, at least, very, very similar.

Owing to factors beyond our control, at our births, Kenny Dalglish was and I was not a potentially great footballer yet, it would be bizarre of me to claim that regarding the distribution of football-playing talents I have been treated inequitably. Perhaps I have been unlucky but that is a different matter. Suppose that a tyrant in some society economically very much less developed than our own decided independently of the choices and wishes of the people to install, in the interest of public health, a public sewerage system. The decision and its implementation need not be inequitable no matter that tyranny, as a general thing, is inequitable and no matter whether or not the undertaker is thereby disadvantaged relative to, say, the tailor, due to factors beyond the tailor's and the undertaker's control.

Suppose that, in a liberal democracy, one of the parties which has a chance of forming a government promises lower taxation and lower public expenditure than the party promises and delivers which succeeds in forming a government. Would it be inequitable if, contrary to their expressed wishes as interpretable from their voting choice, those voting for the losing party ended up paying the same amount in taxes as did those who voted for the winning party and, at least by implication, consented to the resultant level of taxation? Surely not. Otherwise liberal democracies must be – as they might be on other grounds – inherently inequitable.

I think that Le Grand's account of equity is unacceptable. I do not believe that he has articulated an applicable principle of equity. But, suppose that he had done. Let us suspend our disbelief in Le Grand's premise and see where his argument leads him.

According to Le Grand: 'If an individual's ill health results from factors beyond his or her control, then the situation is inequitable; if it results from factors within his or her control, then it is equitable'[2]. Le Grand implies that people can choose to smoke or not to smoke and that those who choose to smoke know the health risks they are running. Those who do not voluntarily run the risk of suffering from smoking-related conditions, diseases and illnesses – non-smokers – should not be required to pay towards the associated health care costs. Those who *suffer* from smoking-related conditions and illnesses should not themselves pay the full costs of consequent health care, according to Le Grand. Since not all smokers will suffer from the conditions and illnesses and there is merely a risk and not a certainty that any particular smoker will incur smoking-related health care costs, Le Grand thinks that it follows that it is the group of risk-takers – the smokers – and not merely the cost-incurrers – the smokers who suffer from smoking-related illnesses and conditions – who should, between them, pay the costs of smoking-related health care.

Le Grand argues that health care costs should be met in two sorts of ways, corresponding to his distinction between costs which are the result of risks voluntarily run and other health care costs.

He says that, where people suffer ill health as a result of factors beyond their control'... they should not suffer losses in consequence; hence, they should have treatment free at the point of use and financed by the community'[3]. He claims that: 'In cases where health risks are not obviously identifiable, then everyone is in some sense at equal risk and, therefore, everyone should bear the expected value of the relevant losses'[4]. A uniform tax should, he suggests, finance this sort of expenditure.

Special tax

On the other hand, he says that: 'In addition, if it were established that some activities (such as smoking), did create greater health risks than others, then a special tax should be levied on those activities, at a level sufficient to generate enough revenue to finance the extra treatment costs. Again the special tax would be hypothecated ...'[5].

This is in line with Le Grand's related assertions: first of all that, where activities are voluntarily embraced and have known health risks, everyone who indulges in the activity should bear the associated health care costs whether or not the indulging is injurious to his or her own health and secondly that only those who voluntarily indulge should bear such costs.

Notice here that the element of compulsory taxation, taxation that is involuntary, beyond the control and choice of individual taxpayers raises a question about the internal consistency of Le Grand's *rationale* for his proposed health system. If Le Grand were to be proposing rules for the constitution of a club or some such thing that people could freely choose to join or not to join then the matter would be different; but Le Grand is talking about a non-optional taxation scheme of a (non-optional, in effect) state. To say the least, it is curious to advocate compulsory taxation in order to further equity as defined by Le Grand. It is particularly curious and, on the face of it, particularly paternalistic to force people not to take a risk which they might well have chosen to take, namely the risk of becoming unwell and not receiving all the treatment which might, to good effect, have been directed towards the restoration of their health.

Compulsory taxation, I have no doubt, often is justifiable but it is justifiable on grounds other than what Le Grand thinks of as 'equity' and it is justifiable *as compulsory taxation* rather than as an enforced pre-payment for some particular good or service. To what should people be entitled solely as a consequence of having paid in taxation what it was their due to pay? They should be entitled not to go to jail for tax evasion.

I might here inadvertently have given the impression that I think that indirect taxation such as, say, taxation on tobacco should, somehow, be thought of as voluntary taxation on the grounds that smoking is a voluntary activity. I do not take this view at all. Very few people, I would suppose, choose to smoke and also to pay tobacco duty. Most people who choose to smoke would rather not pay the tobacco duty and pay it because they are coerced into doing so. Those who would choose to pay the tax (if there were any) are also forced to pay it independently of their wills. Choice and control are separate matters. Suppose that there were to be a tax imposed on, say, voting for the Conservative Party or being a woman and that someone tried to justify this tax on the grounds that it was a voluntary tax since people could choose not to vote for the Conservative Party and, since sex change operations are available, people could choose not to remain female. Advocacy of the tax on these grounds might properly be called hypocritical and so too might a similar advocacy of taxation on smoking. I think that Le Grand's proposed specific taxation no less than his proposed general taxation would conflict with his own defence of what he considers to be 'equity'.

Suppose that Nicki is a heavy smoker and a virgin. Suppose that Vicki is a non-smoker and what you might call a heavy non-virgin. According to Le Grand, or, rather, according to my interpretation of his argument, it would be inequitable if Vicki were required to pay any of the smoking-related health care costs incurred by Nicki (or any other smokers) on the grounds that (equity requires that) smokers -and smokers only – as a group should pay the costs of health care which is directed towards the treatment of conditions the risk of whose acquisition knowably is increased by smoking. Whether or not Le Grand's grounds are the grounds of equity – I do not think that he is citing the principle of equity but suppose that he were – it would be inequitable, in the usual sense of the term (as well as in Le Grand's sense) to acquit Vicki of an obligation to pay towards the smoking-related health care costs of Nicki and other smokers and still to insist that Nicki helped to pay for the sex-related health care costs of Vicki and other non-virgins.

Health care surcharge

If equity required that Nicki paid a health care surcharge for being a smoker then it would equally, so it seems to me, require that she received a corresponding rebate for being a virgin. Perhaps you can and should run a private club or a private insurance scheme along principles such as this but, I would suggest, you cannot and should not try so to organise a society or a public health system.

If you do try to organise a society or public health system on the basis of such a principle then you ought at least to apply the principle consistently and generally. To pick on merely, say, smokers would be unjust, unfair and inequitable.

Smokers and virgins are people and ought to be treated as individual people rather than merely as members of particular groups. If people who are smokers are treated as smokers rather than as individual people, then they should also simultaneously be treated as members or non-members of *all* the other health-risk categories which there are otherwise they will be treated arbitrarily and, in the usual sense of the term, inequitably. A system where, arbitrarily, one group of people is given no support in meeting the costs of the health care which their risk has brought about and is simultaneously forced to help to meet the health care costs which are brought about by the voluntary and knowably risky behaviour of other people seems to me to be manifestly unjust (whatever other merits it might have). Hence, if you want to discriminate against smokers with regard to health care costs and you want to discriminate on the grounds of equity, then make sure that you also discriminate against non-virgins and all other risk-taking and risk-creating groups. Le Grand explicitly states that we should discriminate against all such groups but, given that there are so many of them to choose from, it is perturbing that he refers so often to smokers. What about, say, motorists, drinkers, carnivores and those who take insufficient exercise?

'Passive worrying'

Le Grand's proposal is a dangerous one because, while it is clear that the partial and arbitrary application of his principle will be unfair, unjust and inequitable, it is equally clear that the impartial and consistent application of his principle would not be, for various economic and political reasons, a feasible proposition. For instance, while smoking can be readily monitored, quantified and taxed, other relevant activities (and the lack of them) cannot. Think, say, about the failure to take adequate exercise. Think about worry – a dreadfully unhealthy activity. Think about sex! In addition, while there seems to be votes in the distasteful practice of baiting smokers, there would presumably be none in trying to penalise financially, say, non-virgins and worriers. Through the company of over-anxious, stressed and stressful friends and colleagues, how many of us are the victims of 'passive worrying'? Worrying – so my own experiences of relaxation therapy and of nicotine addiction suggest – is, with proper instruction (which is available within the NHS) no more difficult to give up than smoking is. Or, it can be.

Suppose it were to be announced that, as from, say, next week, the health care costs relating to activity Q – and the health care costs relating only to Q: the health care costs relating to activities R, S, T, U ... Z will be financed from general taxation – will be borne solely by those who indulge in Q. Depending upon what activity Q were – playing tennis?; hill-walking? – there might be a public outcry. Whatever Q were, including smoking or having sex, there ought to be, I am suggesting, an outcry on the basis of fairness, justice and equity. If there were no National Health Service; if there were no compulsory financing of the health care of others; if all health care payments were voluntary then the situation might be quite different.

Suppose that Nicki, the smoker and virgin, will develop and die from lung cancer. Suppose that this will occur under a Le Grand-inspired regime. Given that the cost of Nicki's smoking-related health care will have been pre-paid compulsorily by Nicki and her fellow-smokers then, unlike under the National Health Systems as it currently prevails, Nicki will have a moral right and should have a legal right to the treatment she needs. Non-smokers, please be prepared to stand aside for her! What if she decides to forego medical treatment or to forego all but the most rudimentary sort of it? In these circumstances, since her treatment would have been previously paid for, I think that she would have a case for demanding a cash rebate in lieu of the requisite treatment. Otherwise, would she not be treated (in a different sense of the term) unjustly, unfairly? Would she not be being ripped off by the Le Grand system of 'equitable' health care?

Similarly, given her smoking-related illness, there are costs, including health care costs which she will be unable to impose or, at least, be far less likely to impose on the community than she would have been able to had she not smoked. For instance, Nicki, let us assume, will not receive an old age pension; she will not suffer from nor require, at great cost, to be treated for senile dementia; she will receive no sports injuries or consequent treatment for them; she will spare her GP a huge catalogue of consultations as the result of her early death. If Nicki is going to be financially penalised for the costs attendant upon her being a smoker, it would be unfair were she not to receive a rebate, under a Le Grandian system, for the costs which will have been saved as a result of her smoking. If it were to turn out that, overall, smoking and smokers were not a drain on public expenditure but the opposite, would consistent adherence to Le Grand's principles lead one to advocate the public subsidisation of smoking and smokers?

Moral duty

The picture that emerges of a Le Grand-inspired health care system is an interesting although a very curious one. Curious too would be the sort of society of which a Le Grandian health care and health care costs system could form a characteristic part. Indeed, it hardly seems at all like a society of citizens and taxpayers: it seems more like a club or some quasi-voluntary association with a collection of highly self-regarding members. In a normal society, citizens pay taxes as a legal and, in general, a moral duty to support public expenditure in general, where there will only be by accident (if at all) any correspondence or proportion between what an individual taxpayer contributes and what (if anything) he or she receives individually in return. Under Le Grand's scheme, what smokers, for instance, specifically contribute towards the financing of state expenditure sounds more like enforced pre-payment for a specified service rather than normal taxation. With normal taxation, we all p... in the same pot and its contents are distributed without regard to characteristics of the contributors *qua* contributors or the extent of their individual contributions. Does Le Grand think that all public finance and expenditure should take the form which he suggests in relation to health care? If not why not? If one's contribution to the financing of health care costs should vary in relation to one's likely enjoyment of the services provided, then why should not one's contribution to the financing of *all* state expenditure so vary? (Conversely, if one's contribution to state spending in *general* should *not* be based on one's enjoyment of the consumption of the goods and services involved, why should it be in the case of health care costs?) Some people want, for instance, more money spent than others do on defence. Should those of us who think that defence spending is too high receive a tax rebate? Some people benefit more than others from state expenditure on education. Should there be a relationship between the benefits that individual people receive from education and what individual people pay in taxation towards education? Would there be such a relationship in a consistently ordered society in which a Le Grand-inspired health care costs system was at home? I hope that I am able to control my own life and exercise my own choice (or to be sufficiently lucky) such that I do not end up living in such a society.

Motor-cyclists

Le Grand asks the questions:

'Do heavy smokers who contract lung cancer have the same claim, on equity grounds, to resources to restore them to full health (so far as that might be possible) as non-smokers who contract the disease? Are drivers who refuse to put on seat-belts, or motor-cyclists who refuse to wear helmets, entitled to as much compensation in the event of an accident as those who do not take those precautions? More generally, should not those who consciously and voluntarily assume health risks in order to undertake some activity solely of benefit to themselves bear the consequences if these prove adverse' (6)?

Here, several questions – for rhetorical effect? -are run together which would be better separated. The correct answers to them are, I think: yes, smokers do have the same claim; no, such drivers and motor-cyclists should not be entitled to as much compensation (apart from anything else it is not and it should not be illegal to smoke: it is illegal to drive without a seat belt and to ride a motor-cycle minus a helmet) and no, such people should not in particular pay or pay towards their own health costs at least not in Britain while the NHS still persists.

Notice that while the heavy smoker and the non-smoker will, I suggest, *ceteris paribus* have a claim to medical treatment, neither has a *right* to receive the required treatment in the sense that someone or somebody carries a *duty* to provide it. Perhaps both have an equal *right to be considered* for treatment but the outcome of the consideration might, in some cases, be the reasonable judgment that treatment should be withheld. For instance, perhaps both people are so ill that the treatment required would be inordinately expensive and would have very little chance of success. On some occasions a choice might have been made between providing treatment to a non-smoker whose lungs are so badly damaged – whether through his own voluntary and informed actions or not is beside the point – that the chances of successful treatment are slight and providing the treatment to a heavy smoker whose chances of benefiting from the treatment are extremely good. The situation here should not be regarded as being akin to that of a school headmaster or headmistress distributing punishment or praise nor to a court – to refer to Le Grand's curious, in the circumstances, question about the motorist and motor-cyclist – distributing compensation. The smoker here might have a stronger claim than the non-smoker to receive the treatment.

The claim that smokers as a group should pay the costs of smoking-related health care is provocative but unconvincing. Should the costs of treating smoking-related illnesses and conditions be paid solely by smokers while the costs of treating X-related illnesses and conditions, Y-related illnesses and conditions and Z-related illnesses and conditions are not paid solely, respectively, by Xers, Yers and Zers but are paid involuntarily by all people including smokers? At least on the grounds of equity, fairness and justice, one would have to say: no, definitely not. To be fair to Le Grand, it must be stressed that he does not say that it is only smokers as a group who, as a group, should pay for the treatment of the illnesses and conditions which they knowingly run the risk of suffering from: other groups, he says, should be similarly required to do so. Nonetheless, we know that it is not feasible that *all* risk-taking groups ever would be faced with this requirement. We can say with justified confidence that, in Britain at least, there will not be in the imaginable future a tax on, say, sexual intercourse or on failure to take sufficient exercise.

A very curious society

Even if, somehow, Le Grand's principle of the payment of health-care costs could be applied consistently and equitably, he gives no convincing argument to suggest that it should be. The sort of society where it were consistently applied would seem to be – insofar as one can imagine it – a very curious one. What other curious features would the society need to possess in order to allow for the consistent applications of Le Grand's principle? Should the health care costs pertaining to all *particular* – thereby by addition to *all* – knowably avoidable illnesses and conditions be paid solely by those who run the risk of suffering from *particular* knowably avoidable illnesses and conditions? No, I do not think so. More attractive or, at least, less unattractive would be the principle that: the health care costs pertaining to *all* knowably avoidable illnesses and conditions (just like the rest of them) should be paid by those who voluntarily run the risk of suffering from *any* knowably avoidable illness or conditions -which would seem to be any of us who live and breathe ... or ride in motor cars and/or are pedestrians ... or eat... or have sex ....

*By Hugh V. McLachlan, from the *Journal of Medical Ethics*, 1995, Vol. 21, No. 4, pp. 209-213. Reproduced with permission from the BMJ publishing group.

References

(1) Grand J. *Equity and choice: an essay in economics and applied philosophy.* London: Harper Collins Academic, 1991: 176.

(2) See reference (1): 114.

(3) See reference (1): 124.

(4) See reference (1): 125.

(5) See reference (1): 123.

(6) See reference (1): 113-114.

Chapter Twenty-one

Tobacco Taxation and Fairness*

Smith and Bopp attack what they consider to be my views on taxation and smoking as expressed in a previous article in the *Journal of Medical Ethics*. I shall restate and defend my position. Some problems with Smith's and Bopp's defence of taxation on tobacco as: "... a means of covering the added health care expenses *caused* by smokers' exercise of choice" will then be suggested.[1] In addition, I want to move the debate about the taxation of tobacco forward by questioning the meaning and significance of fairness in this context. Smith and Bopp might well give their readers the impression that I am against the heavy taxation of tobacco. I am not. Often with public policy, what matters is why what is done is done and not merely what is done.

Smokers, Virgins, Equity and Health Care Costs

First of all, let us consider my original position. What is at issue centrally is a philosophical principle of taxation presented by Le Grand: the taxation of tobacco in particular was discussed in my article as being illustrative of the principle concerned.[2] It is Le Grand's contention that, on the grounds of equity, the group of people who voluntarily indulge in what are known to be risky activities (and this group exclusively) should pay through hypothecated taxation for the costs of the health care which that activity causes the need for.[3]

I argued against this. The principle is, I suggested, inherently not particularly equitable. Furthermore, it is not a principle which could, partly for reasons of political practicality, be consistently and equitably applied. The principle that people — individually or collectively — should pay the costs that their voluntary actions occasion might be an appropriate one to apply in some contexts and some types of social organisations, particularly where membership and participation are optional and voluntary. However, in societies, especially in a society such as Britain where health care is provided by the National Health Service (NHS) and funded by taxation, it is not an equitable one — nor on other obvious grounds a suitable one — to apply in relation to health care.

In Britain, would it be equitable were non-virgins and non-virgins alone required to pay for all the costs of the treatment of sexually related illnesses and conditions such as, for instance, venereal disease and pregnancy? No, I do not think that it would be particularly equitable. Non-virgins should not be required to pay more than virgins in taxation in order to cover the health care costs which they, through their voluntary actions, cause. Similarly, I do not think that it would be particularly equitable to require smokers to foot exclusively the bill for smoking-related health care costs. Furthermore it would be inequitable were smokers and smokers alone required to pay for the treatment of smoking-related illnesses while they were also forced, whether or not they were, say, joggers, motorists, drinkers, or virgins, to pay via taxation for jogging, motoring, drinking, and sex-related health care.

Smith and Bopp are right when they say: "Hugh V McLachlan has argued that it is unfair to tax smokers, and smokers alone for the health-related costs associated with smoking".[1] I did not argue, however, against the taxation, even the very high taxation of tobacco: I argued against a particular principle for justifying it.

Smith and Bopp say: "Taxing smokers is sound public policy" and they also say that this taxation is justified as "... a means of covering the added health care expenses caused by smokers' exercise of choice".[1] Taxing the purchase of tobacco — strictly speaking, there is no tax on smoking nor on smokers — is, I agree, sound public policy. It does not, however, require the defence which Smith and Bopp try to give it. There are taxes on, for instance, the purchase of television sets, socks, chocolates, perfume, and beer. The justification for these taxes — and this is typical of taxation in general: why should the taxation of tobacco be different? — is not and need not be that it covers the costs of the health care which is necessitated as a consequence of the effects of, respectively, watching television, wearing socks, eating chocolate, wearing perfume, and drinking beer. To say that there is a justification for a tax on the purchase of commodity X is not the same thing as saying that all health care costs pertaining to illnesses stemming from the consumption of X should be paid for solely by the consumers of X.

Smith and Bopp on Le Grand and McLachlan

Smith and Bopp write: "Both McLachlan and Le Grand presume that smoking is a private vice, based upon informed choice, and that the full costs of smoking are visited upon smokers (and smokers alone)".[1] What an astonishing claim! I presumed in the article no such things (and nor, in his book, does Le Grand). I do not think that the direct and indirect consequences of smoking affect only smokers any more than that the consequences of the actions of non-virgins are visited upon non-virgins alone.

Smith and Bopp say: "Unfortunately, McLachlan's position is based upon a misrepresentation of Le Grand".[1] I do not fully specify Le Grand's position but I do so fully enough for the argument that I make. I give a fair and true account of as much of Le Grand's theory of equity and taxation as is required to be given for a consideration of his argument. Readers can check and decide for themselves whether Bopp and Smith are correct on this point or I am.

Smith and Bopp say: "McLachlan's final criticism amounts to a simple argument from slippery slope — adopting an excise tax on smoking would result in a plethora of special taxes".[1] Slippery slopes have nothing to do with my case. I do not argue that a tax on tobacco will lead to other taxes. I talk of smokers, virgins, non-smokers, and non-virgins but I do not expect or suggest that there will be a tax introduced on sexual intercourse.

The Hypothecated Taxation of Tobacco

Smith and Bopp do not fully specify how they think that a hypothecated tax on tobacco should operate (and nor, to my knowledge, does Le Grand). Should taxation on the current purchase of tobacco pay for: A) the costs of current smoking-related health care or: B) the future smoking-related health care costs of current smokers? There are severe — perhaps insurmountable — problems either way.

For instance, if you choose B), then you have the problem of guessing — you cannot know — what the future health care costs will amount to in order to set a rate of taxation which will cover and will do no more than only cover that amount. What, for instance, will the absolute and relative pay of nurses be in the future? What, if any, relevant and presently unknown medical treatments and techniques will become available in the future? How much will they cost?

If you choose A), then among the problems raised is this one. It might turn out that in the future, fewer and fewer people will smoke and that it will not be possible to raise from the future taxation of tobacco enough money to pay for the treatment of those people who currently smoke and will become ill in the future.

Whether you choose A or B, if the rate of taxation of tobacco in the UK is significantly higher than the rate of taxation of tobacco in other countries then some or many people in the UK will evade the UK tax through the buying of smuggled cigarettes.

The Costs of Smoking

The question of the precise net costs of smoking and of the net costs of smoking borne by non-smokers is crucial for Bopp's and Smith's argument. They do not give an account, however, of what such costs are and nor do they seem to be aware of the complexity of the problem of calculating them.

There is a possibility, perhaps even a likelihood, that, in Britain, smokers as a group subsidise non-smokers as a group. A strict application of the principle advocated by Smith and Bopp might even require a negative tax on — that is, a subsidisation of — the purchase of tobacco. I would be against that. What would Smith and Bopp say?

It is indicated in a recent research note that the costs to the NHS of deaths through smoking of smokers is estimated to be only £1.7 billion while the expected tax revenue from tobacco next year is £7.8 billion.[4] Furthermore, those who die from smoking would not, were they to have been non-smokers, have been immortal. They would have died from other causes and suffered from other costly illnesses.

Why consider only health care costs? There are various other relevant items of public expenditure: in particular, since smokers, on average, do not live as long as non-smokers, they do not as a group generate the same pension costs as non-smokers as a group.

Justice, Fairness and Taxation

The crucial mistake which Smith and Bopp make is to conflate and confuse the two following separate questions. Is an excise tax on tobacco a good tax? Is an excise tax on tobacco a fair tax? It is, in my view, not a fair tax but it is a good one. Let me elaborate on "fairness" and on taxation in order to support this paradoxical claim.

I think it is useful to distinguish between "fairness" and "justice". I think that the notion of fairness is an important one but I do not think that it can be analysed. I suspect that it can be defined, if at all, only ostensibly by giving examples of what we think would count as instances of fairness and of unfairness. What counts as fairness too depends, I think, very much on the particular vantage point from we choose to view situations. There is, in my understanding and preferred use of the term, a relationship between justice and rights which does not exist between fairness and rights or between luck and rights. For instance, I would say that while the deaths of Buddy Holly and John Lennon were both unlucky and unfair, the death of the latter was also unjust.[5,6]

Buddy Holly died in a plane crash as the result of an accidental error of the pilot, who also died. John Lennon was deliberately murdered. Buddy Holly's death was not an infringement of his rights. We do not have a right not to die. The pilot was not in breach of a duty which he had towards Buddy Holly. We do not have a duty not to make mistakes although we have a duty to try not to make them. John Lennon was denied the enjoyment of a right when he died, the right not to be killed.

With some things, if you cannot do them fairly, then you should not do them at all. With other things, if you cannot do them fairly, then you should do them non-fairly or even unfairly. For instance, if you cannot give someone a fair trial on, say, a murder charge, then you should not give him or her a trial at all. On the other hand, suppose you need, in a dire emergency and for a just war, to raise an army. If you cannot raise the army in a fair way, then you should raise it in a non-fair way or even an unfair way: what matters is that you raise it. Raising taxes is akin to the raising (in some peculiar circumstances) of armies: that they are raised is — but that they are raised fairly is not — crucial.

Taxation, as the means of provision of public finance, is necessary for the survival of the state and of society itself in an advanced industrial context. Furthermore, taxation also funds the provision of goods and services which, even if not essential, are useful. It is in relation to such societal survival and usefulness that taxation is justifiable. It is not clear that the provision of such goods and services or even societal survival itself would be possible on the basis *solely* of taxation which was fair. No industrial society, I would suggest, has been known to levy only fair taxes. It is not even clear what fair taxation would consist in. Taxes need not be fair in order to be justifiable.

I would suggest that a poll tax is the fairest (or least unfair) of taxes. It is also one of the worst. The introduction of the Poll Tax was perhaps Mrs Thatcher's major political error. The problem with the Poll Tax in Britain was not that it was unfair or particularly so but that it was, whether rightly or wrongly, *thought to be unfair* and, more importantly that it was *very difficult and expensive to collect*: also, in the incompleteness of it, its (partial) collection was unjust and unfair. It was a bad tax, a very bad tax.

Conversely, although it is unfair (or, at least, not fair) heavy taxation on tobacco is *thought* to be fair: it can be raised without a public outcry. Furthermore, the tax is easy and cheap to collect. The whole point of taxation is to raise money: taxation on tobacco does this bounteously. Excise duty on tobacco is a good tax.

Paternalism

Smith and Bopp say that heavy taxation of tobacco can also be justified on paternalistic grounds. I disagree for two reasons. Paternalism as such is, in general, a poor basis for public policy. Secondly, the taxation of tobacco which is paid by actual smokers — as opposed to the disincentive effect on non-smokers caused by the existence of tax on tobacco — is not an instance of paternalism. The beneficiaries of the policy are, by definition, not smokers. You benefit from the tax only to the extent that you don't pay it. To penalise individual X for the benefit of X is – whether justified or not — paternalism. To tax individual Y for the benefit of X is not — whether justified or not — paternalism: it is, or is more like, authoritarianism.

Conclusion

My position can withstand the criticism of Smith and Bopp. An excise duty on tobacco can be defended but (at least in contemporary Britain) not on the grounds of fairness and/or equity as "...a means of covering the added health care expenses caused by smokers' exercise of choice" despite what Smith and Bopp and Le Grand say. The taxation, indeed, the heavy taxation of tobacco is justifiable but it is justifiable despite its unfairness (or, perhaps, non-fairness) rather than because it is particularly fair or equitable.

*By Hugh V McLachlan, from the *Journal of Medical Ethics*, 2002, Vol. 28 No. 6, pp. 381-383. Reproduced with permission from the BMJ publishing group.

References

1. Smith VR, Bopp AE. Smokers and taxes. *Journal of Medical Ethics* 1999;25:419. Medline
2. McLachlan HV. Smokers, virgins, equity and health care costs. *Journal of Medical Ethics* 1995;21:209–13. Medline
3. Le Grand J. *Equity and choice: an essay in economics and applied philosophy*. London: Harper Collins Academic, 1991.
4. Davis C. Findings. *The Times Higher Education Supplement* 2002

Jan 11: 8.
5. McLachlan HV. Justice, rights and health care: a discussion of the Report of the Commission on Social Justice. *International Journal of Sociology and Social Policy* 1998;18:65–84.
6. McLachlan HV. Scotland, social justice, health and inequality. In: Nottingham C, ed. *The NHS in Scotland: the legacy of the past and the prospect of the future*. Aldershot: Ashgate, 2000: 106–23.

Chapter Twenty-two

Justice and the NHS: A Comment on Culyer*

Abstract

The nature and significance of equity and equality in relation to health and healthcare policy is discussed in the light of a recent article by Culyer.[1] Culyer makes the following claims: (a) the importance of equity in relation to the provision of health care derives from the human need for health in order to flourish; and (b) for the sake of equity, equality of health among the members of particular political jurisdictions should be the aim of health policy. Both these claims are challenged in this paper. The argument put forward is that it is only when needs arise and are met in particular contexts that need and equity are fused. The state and its agents and agencies should distribute what it distributes impartially, whatever it distributes. Whether or not equity applies to the distribution of healthcare services depends on now they are provided and not on their nature as "primary goods". Contrary to what Culyer suggests, a policy of trying to produce the outcome of health equality would be inequitable. It would not be impartial and it would fail to treat persons as persons ought to be treated.

Introduction

In his account of equity and health care, Culyer makes the following two broad claims:

- the importance of equity in relation to the provision of health care derives from the human need for health in order to flourish.
- for the sake of equity, equality of health among the members of particular political jurisdictions should be the aim of health policy.

Both claims will be challenged in this paper.

Equity, Justice, and Impartiality

Of equity in general, Culyer writes:

'In essence all equity approaches judge the treatment of individuals inequitable if it is capricious or relates to "irrelevant" characteristics .... Equity in health care requires that patients who are alike in relevant respects be treated in like fashion and that patients who are unlike in relevant respects be treated in appropriately unlike fashion.'[2]

I go along with Scruton's view that, other than in a peculiar legal sense of the term, "[e]quity is another name for just dealing"[3] Culyer seems to me to be referring to a particular instance of the general principle of justice that people and agencies should do what they have a duty to do and should be given that which they have a right to receive.[4] It is, in some contexts, a matter of justice or "equity" that people are treated impartially; that is to say, in some, although not all contexts, some people have a right to be treated impartially and other particular people and agencies have a duty to mete out such treatment.

Impartiality as such is not a virtue. It assumes its morally laudable nature in the context of rights and duties. Furthermore, impartiality in relation to equity is something more than and other than the mere consistent application of rules of behaviour. Actions, in order to be good ones must treat persons appropriately as persons. This is the bedrock of all good actions and, therefore, of all good just actions.

A man who treats his own wife and his neighbour's wife impartially when it comes to the distribution of, say, his pay and his sexual attentions, would be treating his wife inequitably. The same man, were he to be, for instance, a judge or a university lecturer would be required, when acting *qua* judge or lecturer to treat all convicted felons and students who came before him as such (including his own and his neighbour's wife) impartially. Where a relevant reason exists for treating them differently, then he must discriminate between them; otherwise he must not do so in any significant way. If an unmarried judge or university lecturer is, in his capacity as a private citizen, choosing a casual sexual partner or choosing people to invite to a party he is throwing, then he is not required by equity to treat people impartially. No one has a right to be invited to his party or a right to his sexual favours: he can distribute his invitations and his sexual favours partially and without any justification for favouritism without acting inequitably.

The Yorkshire Ripper was not impartial in his choice of murder victims. He chose only women. However, had he been "an equal opportunities" slaughterer and killed men and women indiscriminately, his actions would have been no less wicked and no less inequitable. Equity involves not merely the relevantly equal treatment of persons but the treatment, equally and indiscriminately, of persons as persons ought to be treated. The recent writings of Levine capture this notion well. He writes that: "Dueness, fairness and impartiality all entail a kind of equality, the kind associated with equal regard for personhood".[5]

Dworkin's Egalitarian Objection to Culyer's Egalitarianism

According to Dworkin:

"No government is legitimate that does not show equal concern for the fate of all those over whom it claims dominion and from whom it claims allegiance. Equal concern is the sovereign virtue of political community — without it government is only tyranny. ..".[6]

This is an interesting formulation of the issue whether or not it is completely satisfactory. Governments should treat citizens impartially but not, in my view, because they should be equally concerned about them. Whatever the nature and extent of their concern, that is what they are obliged to do. Mention of the "fate" of individual citizens is curious and would seem to be unnecessary. If we treat people properly and, thereby, show appropriate concern for individual persons as persons, we have done enough: concern for the fates of the people concerned is not an additional requirement.

Dworkin shows that equality of resources is not the same as — nor will it lead to — equality of welfare. As an egalitarian, he argues for equality of resources rather than of welfare. He presents the following argument against any sort of advocacy of equality of welfare, of which Culyer's argument is an instance. Different people will have different preferences for different sorts of good things including, we can say, health and health care. Dworkin contends that: "people cannot be treated as equals by making them equal in some dimension they value unequally...".[7] It is not clear how Culyer would respond to the objection that there is an arbitrariness and unfairness about his selection of health as that which should be equalised.

By way of a possible illustration and adaptation of Dworkin's point, imagine four members of a community and suppose that they were all equally healthy partly as a consequence of the public spending on health care. One of them, let us suppose, would rather be better educated than he was and prefer to have less money spent on health care and more on education even if he were in consequence less healthy. Another might prefer to be better defended against external attack even if, as a consequence, fewer resources are devoted to education and/or health care. The third might prefer to devote more resources to charitable foreign aid and/or to savings and investments for the sake of the wellbeing of her grandchildren even if, as a consequence, her health, although good, was not as good as it might have been. The fourth would prefer to live a shorter but a more prosperous life and pay less in taxes and have more money in her own pockets. To insist, come what may, on a policy of equal health, as Culyer appears to do, would be to disregard the essential personhood of those who would benefit or suffer from the implementation of it.

Why, if, and when it does, does Equity Matter?

Culyer raises the question: "Why be concerned about equity in health care distribution?".[2] According to him, equity is of importance in relation to healthcare provision because of the nature and significance of health and health care. The distribution of health care, or so he argues, is and should be thought of as being different from the distribution of normal goods and services. It is Culyer's view that: "Entities such as health derive equity significance from their ability to enable people to 'flourish'".[2] Culyer writes:

'What is this particular significance about health that raises its status in equity above other services? The answer seems to be that health, like the cognitive skills developed by educational institutions, is one of a special set of characteristics (sometimes called "primary goods") about whose distribution people are particularly concerned .... Aristotle termed this concept "eudaemonia", which is usually taken to mean "flourishing".'[2]

I would argue that, if the state provides a good or service then, whether or not there is a need for it and whether or not it leads to human flourishing, the state should distribute it equitably because the state and its agents and agencies have a duty to treat citizens impartially and they have a corresponding right to impartial treatment. Where the state does not, directly or indirectly, provide the good or service, considerations of equity do not necessarily apply in the same way even if the good or service is needed for human flourishing.[8,9]

Consider the latter point first. Among the things that I require in order to flourish, in order, even, to live are, for instance: food, blood, water and oxygen. In order to flourish and not to languish, I need, for instance, music, literature, religion, and sex. It does not, as a matter of logic, follow that, because I and other people need these things, the state should provide them for us. Whether it would be a good idea to have a system whereby the state provided any or all of these requirements would depend on factors other than our need for them. There will be advantages and disadvantages of the state provision of particular goods and services in different circumstances. For instance, some conditions such as plagues, famines, earthquakes, or wars can make the case for the state rationing and direct provision of foodstuffs morally, politically, and economically compelling. We need food no less in normal conditions where such state distribution, however equitable, would be far worse than a non-equitable plenitude. Without oxygen I will very quickly die. However, a system where I depended on the state for the provision of such oxygen that I need would, even if a practical possibility, be hellish. Perhaps at some time in the future there will be a National Oxygen Service and people will need to use it. Then, the state would be obliged to distribute oxygen equitably. It is only when needs arise and are met in particular contexts that need and equity are fused.

Some of the things that the state and its agents distribute are more important then others. Some are literally a matter of life and death whereas others are trivial. The duty to act impartially holds throughout. For instance, consider state lotteries. Whether the prize is several million pounds or a ten pound note, there is a right to impartial treatment held by the participants and a corresponding duty of impartiality borne by those who run the lottery. In all actions where a difference of treatment of the individuals who officially come before them involves a difference in benefit or burden to these individuals then the agents and agencies have a duty to act impartially and the individuals have a right to receive impartial treatment. Of course, some infractions of the duty of impartiality are more heinous than others. Sometimes, too, considerations other than that of equity make some inequitable actions more or less blameworthy than they would otherwise be.

When the National Health Service (NHS) distributes health care then it has, as a duty to act impartially, a duty to treat (in the non-medical sense) those who have claims on their services impartially. In comparison with matters of life and death, some – perhaps most – of the services which the NHS has to offer are trivial. However, it is obliged to distribute them, no less than the others, impartially. It would be no less inequitable to distribute, for example, bedpans than heart transplants on the basis, say, of the political views of the claimants although it would be on other grounds a more serious inequitable action. Consider an analogy: in one sense, it is far worse to steal £1000 than to steal £5 but, in another sense, it is the quality of the action – the nature of it rather than its quantifiable aspect – wherein lies its wrongness.

People can have legal and moral rights to things that they do not need nor want. For instance, the suicidal and the terminally ill have, no less than anyone else, moral and legal rights not to be killed. If I borrow a five pound note from Bill Gates, he has a moral and a legal right to its recovery whether or not he needs or wants it. Hence, Culyer is, I think, mistaken when he says: "equity requires that services go only to those who need them...".[10] Culyer is, similarly, mistaken, I suggest, when he says: "Health care that is not related to the protection, promotion, and restoration of health may have ample justification in terms of the satisfaction of consumed preferences, but it is not to be evaluated by equity criteria".[11] The state, its agents, and agencies should distribute what it distributes impartially, whatever it distributes.

When I was a young schoolboy at Paisley Grammar School, I was one of the few pupils in my class to be presented with a splendid tin-box full of sweets. This was to celebrate a particular anniversary pertaining to Johnstone, a nearby town I then lived in. The local council in Johnstone was not obliged by equity to distribute sweets to schoolchildren. However, if they decided, for whatever reason, to distribute sweets, they were obliged to distribute them impartially. I did not need, although I very much enjoyed and appreciated, the sweets. Conversely, even though we might need, say, food, sex, religion, or health care to flourish it does not follow that such things must, as a matter of equity, be provided by the state.

Does Health Inequality Matter? If so, why does it?

It is Culyer's contention that: "An equitable health care policy should seek to reduce the inequality in health (life expectation, self-reported morbidity, quality of life in terms of personal and social functioning) at every stage of the life cycle".[2] He continues[12]:

'Such a policy must meet needs, but in proportion to the "distance" each individual is from the population average ... the principle underlying the selection of needs to be met will not be a simple, proportionate one in terms of needs. Instead, needs will be met so as to reduce the dispersion of ill health in the community.'

I would claim that, contrary to what Culyer suggests, a policy of trying to produce the outcome of health equality would be inequitable, however much it might be – if it is – defensible on other moral grounds. Not all morally good outcomes are morally appropriate targets. Not all morally appropriate targets are justified by equity.

Suppose several people request particular books from their local public library and that not all of the requests can be acceded to. Say, in the first instance, that, with the intention of treating each individual requester impartially and fairly, on the basis of "first come first served", particular books are given to particular people. Consider next an alternative distributional policy whereby books are distributed with the intention of trying to reduce inequalities in erudition among members of and groups in the local community. With the operation of this alternative policy, it is quite likely that if the same people had made the same requests for books, the distribution of the books would have been different: other books, in all likelihood, would have been given to other people. Even if it turned out by a curious chance that both policies had the same outcome and that under both policies, the same books would have been distributed to the same people, the second policy, unlike the first one would not have been equitable. Equity relates not merely to what is done to people but why and how it is done. The second policy does not consider individual people with fairness and with appropriate and equal respect as individual people: it considers them as means towards the realisation of the egalitarian vision of the policy maker. The library staff have a duty to treat the library users as individuals in their own right. The alternative policy is in breach of that duty. It is also directed to an aim that it is not the business of librarians *qua* librarians to pursue. In their spare time, librarians, doctors, hospital managers, members of parliament, and prime ministers can try to realise their moral visions; when they are acting in their official capacities, there are constraints on what they are permitted and required to do.

Similarly, suppose people were to be given and denied particular medical treatment provided by the state, not on the basis of their individual requests as individual people but, alternatively, on the basis of the intended outcome of such treatment with reference to the inequalities of health within the communities of which they are members. Such a policy would be inequitable; it would be a breach of the principle of impartiality. The different medical treatment given to different people would not relate to relevant differences between the people themselves but to the egalitarian whim of the policy maker. Furthermore, the people would not have been treated appropriately as individual persons. Even if the actual medical treatment given and denied to particular individuals would, in some circumstances or other, be the same under the operation of both policies, the latter policy would, I suggest, still be inequitable because of how and why it was done. The latter policy and its outcomes might, of course, be justifiable but if they were, they would be justified by grounds and virtues other than equity.

Culyer's Policy Proposals and Mine in Practice

If three people request major heart surgery and another three people request treatment for in-growing toenails, under the NHS or a similar state funded healthcare system, in what order should the people be allocated treatment? In my view, an equitable procedure would be to allocate what treatment was available on a first come first served basis. However, equity alone cannot determine what health care should be available and how it should be distributed. Equity rules out rather than specifies particular courses of action.

Does it matter whether or not the prospective patients need the treatment and how much they need it? For reasons other than equity – for instance, consequentialist concerns about the increase of happiness and the decrease of pain and also, say, public perceptions of fairness – we might make it a rule of the NHS that citizens must need what treatment they request in order to be considered eligible for it. Similarly, we could make it a rule that no NHS resources are devoted to medically minor matters such as in-growing toenails while there are patients who need more medically important treatment such as major heart surgery. Equity does not require that patients are treated on the basis of need. However, treatment on the basis of the needs of patients as individuals is not inconsistent with equity: it is not necessarily inequitable.

Suppose that of the people seeking heart surgery, one of them lives in a multiply deprived area of Glasgow and another is a member of an ethnic minority and that, of those seeking treatment for their feet, one is unemployed and another is a single parent. In my view, this information is irrelevant for the equitable allocation of health care. Culyer's approach is quite different. According to Culyer, "What ought to dominate is *the distribution of health* and how health care interventions can alter that for the better".[12] Policymakers and implementers, according to Culyer, require to act upon:

"Information on the current distribution of resources and health (or sickness) in relation to 'target groups' [that is social categories of people with particular propensities for ill-health] and any other groups perceived as ethically significant..."

and to make:

"Informed judgements about the effect of changes in resource distribution on the health of individuals and especially target groups".[13]

Culyer says that policy makers should take into account and be aware of certain things for the sake of equity that I say, for the sake of equity, they should ignore. He says that, for the sake of equity, the allocation of health care should be directed to particular social categories, geographical areas and "target groups": I say that, for equity's sake it should be directed to individual citizens *qua* individual citizens.

What is Done and What Happens

Culyer runs a number of curious claims together when he says[2]:

'If it is felt that all residents of a political jurisdiction ought to have equal opportunities for their lives to flourish, then it follows that health care is one of those goods and services whose right distribution must be ensured.'

What Culyer says follows does not follow at all. Culyer is here conflating quite different questions[14]: What, were it to happen, would be a good outcome? What ought to be done? Who ought to do it?[15] Even if it is the case (which one might dispute) that it would be good, were it to happen, that all residents of a political jurisdiction had equal opportunities for their lives to flourish, it does not follow that you, we, the Prime Minister, or the NHS or the government (or anyone or anything) should act in such a way as to bring that state of affairs about. Our obligations might well pull us towards other courses of action.

Even if he is correct in assuming that it would be good if all residents of a community had the sort of opportunities which Culyer talks of here, it certainly does not follow that the state should regulate the distribution of health care – far less the distribution of health – in the way that Culyer advocates. If the state provides health care then that health care should be distributed impartially by the state. If health and ill health are unequally distributed, even as a partial consequence of this equitable treatment, so be it. The state is responsible for its actions and has an obligation to try to ensure that its actions are just. It is not obliged to ensure that the outcome of its actions, in combination with a host of other factors, will produce a fair, or in any other respect a morally desirable distribution of health. The distribution of health is not the business of the state, or of its agents or agencies. The state (and its agents and agencies) is not responsible for what turns out to be people's portion of health. The state, like the rest of us must, as a prerequisite of justice, mind its own business.

In relation to fairness, equity, and justice, the state is required to act fairly, equitably, and justly: it is not required to ensure or to try to ensure that its acts – in conjunction with a host of other factors beyond its control and responsibility – produce fair, equitable, and just outcomes.

Conclusion

Both of Culyer's claims about equity and health care are dubious. The importance of equity in relation to the provision of health care does not spring from the human need for health. The equalisation of health is not an equitable aim of public policy. So I have argued.

Health care – like formal education but unlike health and erudition, which are not transferable – can be considered in economic terms as a "good" or service. Culyer talks of "primary goods" in this context and in so doing he refers to Tobin and alludes to Rawls.[16,17] Primary goods for these writers are regarded as fundamentally necessary for the good life; they are needed by all for flourishing. It is, of course, morally good that such needs (if there are such needs) are met and that such goods (if such there are) are provided but it is not necessarily a matter of equity that they are provided. Whether or not equity applies to their distribution depends on how they are provided and not on their nature as primary goods. It is not necessarily appropriate that they are provided by the state. It is not a matter of equity that they are provided by the state. However, if they are provided by the state they should be distributed equitably.

There is a distinction between equality of treatment and equality of outcome. Similarly, equitable treatment is not the same as "equitable outcome", if this is an intelligible notion. Outcomes can be morally appraised but it is not clear that they can be either equitable or inequitable. The crucial point is this. We are responsible for what we do: we are not similarly responsible for the outcome in its entirety of what we do. The state cannot control and it has no responsibility for the distribution of, say, erudition and health in general: rather, it controls and has responsibility for only that formal education and that health care that it provides. It is responsible for providing it equitably. It is not responsible for the outcome of that equitable provision. That outcome will be affected by a host of factors other than that state provision. By analogy, it is the responsibility of, for instance, courts to give all individuals who appear before them impartial, fair, and just treatment. What the outcome of this treatment in conjunction with a batch of other factors and treatment and outcomes will be is not the responsibility of the courts nor is it a matter of equity. If the courts tried to produce what was thought of as a socially equal outcome with, say, as many men and women and white people and non-white people and so forth in prison as their numbers in the population suggested, they would be acting inequitably thereby. Culyer's proposed policy, if it were to be adopted by the NHS, would be no less inequitable even if less heinously so. Of course, to say this is not to say that outcomes do not matter. Politics is not reducible to ethics: ethics is not reducible to the principle of equity. A library service or, say, a health service that had only one virtue would not provide much of a service if that virtue were equity. Other less equitable but busier, cheaper, and less fussy ones might be more satisfactory.

*By Hugh V. McLachlan, from the *Journal of Medical Ethics*, 2005, Vol. 31, No.7, pp. 379-382. Reproduced with permission from the BMJ publishing group.

References

1 Culyer AJ. Equity—some theory and its policy implications. *J Med Ethics* 2001;27:275-83.

2 See reference 1: 276.

3 Scruton R. *A dictionary of political thought* London: Pan Books, 1982:153.

4 See Barry B. *Justice as Impartiality. Vol. II of A Treatise on Social Justice,* Oxford: Clarendon Press, 1995.

5 Levine DP. *Self-seeking and the pursuit of justice.* Aldershot: Ashgate, 1997:3.

6 Dworkin R. *Sovereign virtue:* The *theory and practice of equality.* London: Harvard University Press, 2002:1.

7 See reference 6: 63.

8 See McLachlan HV Justice, rights and health care: a discussion of the report of the Commission on Social Justice. *M J Social Soc Policy* 1998;18:65-84.

9 See McLachlan HV. Scotland, social justice, health and inequality. In: Nottingham C, ed. *The NHS in Scotland: the legacy of the past and the prospect of the future.* Aldershot: Ashgate, 2000:106-23.

10 See reference 1: 280.

11 See reference 1: 277.

12 See reference 1: 281.

13 See reference 1: 282.

14 This conflation is not peculiar to Culyer. It is, for instance, imbedded in utilitarianism and in welfare economics.

15 See McLachlan HV, Swales JK. A drunk driver, a sober pedestrian and the allocation of tragically scarce and indivisible emergency hospital treatment. *Health Care Analysis* 1999,7:5-21.

16 Tobin J. On limiting the domain of inequality. *J Law Econ* 1970;5:263-78.

17 Rawls J. *A Theory of Justice.* Cambridge: Harvard University Press, 1971.

The nature and significance of justice and equity is discussed more fully by McLachlan in *Social Justice, Human Rights and Public Policy*, 2005, Humming Earth, Glasgow.

Posthumous Insemination and Consent

Chapter Twenty-three

Posthumous Insemination and Consent: The Continuing, Troubling Case of Mr and Mrs Blood*

Introduction

In a recent and thoughtful article, Andrew Scott discusses the celebrated case of Diane Blood and the posthumous use of her husband's sperm. We share Scott's uneasiness about the case and about posthumous conception in general. Scott's article leads us to comment on some of the issues that the case raises. Scott asks: 'If Blood occurs again, what should our reaction be ?'[1] We shall offer an answer. Before doing so, however, we shall recount what, so far, has happened.

The Background of the Case: What Happened

Mr and Mrs Blood had been trying to have children in the normal fashion – they were not receiving fertility treatment of any sort – when Mr Blood developed meningitis. He fell into a coma and, at the request of his wife, some of his sperm was removed from him by electro-ejaculation and stored in a licensed clinic, namely, the Jessop Hospital in Sheffield, UK. When Mr Blood died, Mrs Blood requested that the sperm be used to inseminate her. Because the couple had not been receiving fertility treatment, it was required by the Human Fertilisation and Embryology Act 1990 that Mr Blood gave written consent to the use of his sperm. However, Mr Blood had not done so and hence the Human Fertilisation and Embryology Authority (HFEA) refused Mrs Blood permission to use the sperm. It also turned down Mrs Blood's request to have the sperm sent to the Centre for Reproductive Medicine in Brussels, Belgium, which had agreed to inseminate Mrs Blood with Mr Blood's sperm, if it was available. As Scott indicates, in Belgium, '... only verbal evidence of prior consent is required before treatment will be authorised'[2.] So much the worse for Belgium, one might think.

Not only did Mr Blood not give written consent to the use of his sperm, he did not give consent of any sort (whether 'informed' or not) to the treatment which procured it. The defence that the treatment was necessary for his desired and possible recovery was of no avail, since the treatment was carried out only in the expectation that, with or without it, he would die. Had he survived, his testicles would have been, we are led to believe, irreparably damaged. As Fergusson demonstrates, in a very perceptive article in the *Scots Low Times,* not only would the use of the sperm, without Mr Blood's written consent, have been illegal but its seizure was, in itself, illegal. Fergusson writes :

"The Act [i.e. the Human Fertilisation and Embryology Act, 1990] requires written consent to the actual use of the gametes but is silent as to the procedures to be followed when the sample is taken. This does not, of course, mean that there is no requirement for consent at that earlier stage. The common law governs the initial taking of a sample, and clearly a person must consent to this procedure. Any interference with a person without his or her consent is a battery (or in Scots law, an assault). Lord Winston, one of the pioneers of *in vitro* fertilisation, has argued the law does not require written consent for any other medical or surgical procedure, so should not demand written consent for the taking and using of sperm. Although it is true to say that the law does not require written consent to medical treatment, it does however require consent, and the problem with this case is that it seems that the doctors did not even have Mr Blood's oral consent to the taking (let alone the use) of his gametes, since he was in coma at the time" [3].

The case went to judicial review and then to the Court of Appeal. The latter confirmed that the taking and storing of Mr Blood's sperm was, in the absence of his written consent, illegal and that, consequently, any subsequent insemination in Britain would be illegal. However, and very curiously, it suggested that the HFEA might reconsider its decision not to authorise the sending of the sperm to Belgium on the grounds that, under Articles 59 and 60 of the European Community Treaty, Mrs Blood had a right, directly enforceable in English Law, to medical treatment in another Member State. The HFEA reversed its previous decision and authorised the transfer of the sperm.

In our view, it would have been more satisfactory in relation both to the established outcome of this particular case and for the status and reputation of the HFEA had it maintained, more resolutely in the face of intense media pressure and unusual legal decisions, its (very reasonable) original position. Moreover, one suspects that those who are wary about increasing legal integration within the European Union would not have been reassured by this case.

Scott says that there has been no press coverage of the outcome of the treatment. Since the publication of his article, it has been publicised that Mrs Blood's first child, Liam, who was conceived by the posthumous use of Stephen Blood's semen is, at the time of writing, three years of age. Mrs Blood has also just given birth to a second healthy baby in July 2002 in the same Belgian clinic with the same artificial insemination technique using again the sperm of the late Stephen Blood [4]. Mrs Blood was quoted as saying before the birth: "My greatest wish is that the child is born healthy, but an accurate birth certificate would be welcome icing on the cake." [5]

Liam was born three and a half years after the death of his father — his biological but not legal father. On the child's birth certificate, the father is officially stated as 'unknown'. According to the *Herald* newspaper, the UK government has indicated that it will try to change the law so that -unlike the law as it now stands – where sperm is used posthumously, the deceased provider of the sperm ('donor ' is not the correct word here) could be legally designated as the father of the child. The government also said that it would try to make the law retrospectively applicable to 1991.

So far, the government has not found time for the suggested legislation. Perhaps it has changed its mind. It can be anticipated that Mrs Blood will be making strenuous and well-publicised efforts to have the law changed. The leader comment of the *Herald* newspaper on the day of the public announcement of Mrs Blood's second pregnancy was to the effect that there are no matters of importance which require discussion or about which there is room for reasonable disagreement. It says that: "Bureaucrats should not be allowed to deny, or delay any longer, her final wish: her husband's name rightfully on their birth certificates " [6].

Consent

Consent is important. People should be granted a say in what happens to parts of, and issues from, their bodies – not, perhaps, in all circumstances but at least – when the parts or issues are used for the production of their biological offspring. The wishes of the dead should be considered and respected. Furthermore, it can be alarming for the living to think that, after their death and contrary, possibly, to their present wishes, they might become biological parents.

There is a difference between wanting something and consenting to it. To give consent to something can serve to authorise other people to do things which they would not otherwise be entitled to do. The fact that the person wanted the thing to happen and even the fact that he or she said that he or she wanted it to happen does not justify the actions of others in quite the same way. For instance, you can sell your house by consenting to do so but that is not the same as wanting to do so or even the same as saying that you want to do so. Consenting is the saying, under particular circumstances, that what you are doing is consenting to some specific thing or action.

Consent is important in relation to the posthumous use of one's sperm and it is also important that the consent is written. It is important that the person giving consent realises that what he is doing is giving consent and not merely mouthing words. To say, or sing: 'I'd walk a million miles for one of your smiles' is not normally the same as entering into a morally and/or legally binding agreement by virtue of the voluntary giving of consent. It is, usually, the mere mouthing of words. To insist on written consent for the use of sperm can make it clear to the reasonable donor that what he is doing, and what he will be taken to be doing, is giving consent when he gives his consent in writing. His action is not, so he will realise, and will not be taken for something akin to a karaoke performance or, say, for merely the expression of comforting words and thoughts to distressed partners, relatives or friends.

Written consent also serves for the rest of us as good and lasting and citable evidence that consent has been given. It is evidence both that someone went through the motions of giving consent and that he knew – or, at least, should have realised – what these motions signified.

The use of written consent can also help to make it clear to the consenting person and to the rest of us what precisely was consented to. After all, no one would, or, at least, no one should, consent to the unconditional use of his sperm. One should not, for instance, consent to the selling of any consequent babies into slavery or to the use of such babies for the entertainment of torturers. Someone might consent to the use of his sperm for the production of a baby which will be cared for by a stable couple but not for the production of a baby which will knowingly be placed with a single parent even if this parent is the widow of the donor. Another person might consent to the use of his sperm for the production of a baby by his wife or his widow but by no one else.

Is it reasonable to assume that, had he been able to do so, Mr Blood would have consented to the use of his sperm after his death for the possible impregnation of his wife? No, this does not seem to be reasonable. More importantly, in general, it would be quite outrageous to assume that merely because a man consents to marry a woman, it means that the man implicitly consents to father, when dead, her child.

It is now accepted that rape within marriage is possible. In other words, merely because a women has married a particular man, it is no longer generally agreed that consent from that women to have sex with the man can be taken to have been given or be assumed to be implied by the marriage. Given this, it would be bizarre if the assumption were now made that marriage to a woman can give grounds for asserting that the man's consent to the posthumous fathering of her child can reasonably be implied.

Reference to rape is, perhaps, significant here. What is morally and legally pivotal in rape cases is not what a woman might have said or what her wishes were and what she might have consented to (nor, even, what she desired or might have desired) but what she did consent to. Rape is sexual intercourse without consent. Similarly with the case of Mr Blood, what seems crucially important to us is the matter of what, if anything, Mr Blood actually consented to.

Although there is obviously also a practical and a romantic case against it, there might be good reasons for saying that even with normal sexual intercourse, and even, perhaps, within marriage, both parties should be expected to stipulate in writing what precisely they are consenting to. In particular, do they consent to their sperm or eggs being responsible for a pregnancy? Do they consent to intercourse strictly on the understanding that a pregnancy will not result from it?

Even if the use of the sperm could have been legal without Mr Blood's written consent, we would suggest that the illegal manner of its acquisition would be a good reason for saying that its subsequent use to impregnate Mrs Blood should be prohibited. Given that the sperm was procured as a result of assault, its use thereafter should have been restricted even if there were no other legal restrictions on its use. Even apart from any other considerations, encouragement should not be given to possible future similar assaults. It is no use saying that this should not and will not set a precedent. What will be cited as a precedent will be revealed only by future events and decisions. It should be noted, moreover, that the very storage of the sperm without Mr Blood's written consent and not merely its use was illegal.

Although what happened to Mr Blood was not rape, it was something very similar to it. Suppose that a wife were in a coma and that – obviously without her consent – the husband, with the purpose of thereby becoming the father of her child, had sexual intercourse with her. Might not this be rape? Would not it be morally wrong? Suppose that, even more brutally than this, through some sort of electrical treatment, eggs were removed from her body – without her written or any other sort of consent – to be fertilised outside her body to produce, after her death, a baby. Would not there be – and rightly be – a public outcry against such a treatment of the woman? Why should there be such a different reaction to the treatment of a man?

Artificial Insemination and Single and Widowed Women

Mr Blood did not give his consent to the use of his sperm and Mr Blood died. An issue arises directly from his lack of consent. Another arises indirectly from his being dead. In the absence of consent it would be wrong to use Mr Blood's sperm. Even if consent had been given by him for its use in artificial insemination, it would not necessarily be desirable or right for it to be used to inseminate his widow whether he gave specific consent to this or not. Should widows and other single women be given artificial insemination? The identity of the donors is irrelevant to the wisdom of the treatment although not perhaps to its attraction for some of the recipients. Who the donor is and whether he is alive or dead is beside the point here: what matters is that he (the donor) will not act socially as the father of any consequent child nor, as things stand, will any one else.

The Report of the Warnock Commission said that: "The use by a widow of her dead husband's semen for AIH (Artificial Insemination by Husband) is a practice which we feel should be actively discouraged " [7]. We are attracted towards this view although not for the reasons specified in the Report. It says in the Report:

"... we have grave misgivings about AIH (Artificial Insemination by Husband) in one type of situation. A man who has placed his semen in a semen bank may die and his widow may then seek to be inseminated.... This may give rise to profound psychological problems for the child and the mother " [8].

This concern is reflected in Section 13 (5) of the Human Fertilisation and Embryology Act, 1991, which states that:

"A woman shall not be provided with treatment services unless account has been taken of the welfare of any child who may be born as a result of the treatment (including the need of that child for a father)".

It is not clear what force consideration of the interests of the child who may be born can have in this context. It is, surely, better to be born fatherless than not to be born at all, unless one's life is one of peculiarly intense and unusual suffering. However, also worth considering here are the members of society other than the child and the mother, members who, collectively, might be required to support and bear the consequences of this domestic arrangement. Note that conventional social thinking, exemplified by the operation of the Child Support Agency in the UK, is that the supporting of a child is and should be the responsibility of both of its parents. Such bilateral support can scarcely be expected in the case of posthumous insemination.

In the normal way of things, as one would expect, undesirable liaisons are often formed and unfortunate familial outcomes ensue. Often, little can be done about it and it is not practical to try to organise and control private acts of sexual intercourse. However, artificial insemination is not the normal method of conception. It allows the possibility for reflective and public deliberation about its allocation, which could be to a greater extent planned and organised, than normal sexual intercourse could (and should) be. In any case, even with natural insemination, citizens and the state are not always neutral about the domestic and procreative arrangements of people. After all, one might say that while, in many instances, lone parents who become parents as a result of normal sexual intercourse, are good and successful parents and in addition, often, no drain at all on the state's purse, lone parenting, while it certainly should not be illegal, should be discouraged. This should happen even if only through the voicing of the opinion that, in general, joint parenting is preferable.

Medical Treatment

We are very much in agreement with the views of McHale, Fox and Murphy when they say:

"It remains to be seen whether the Court of Appeal is correct in its view that its decision sets no precedent for future cases. It is also significant that an issue raising fundamental questions about the significance of informed consent, reproductive autonomy and the status of gametes was transposed into the context of freedom to avail of services " [9].

To say that Mrs Blood has a 'right' – of whatever sort – to treatment in, for instance, a clinic in Belgium is one thing, but to say that she has a rightful claim to the use of her dead husband's sperm for that particular treatment, would seem to us to be something else. She can have the treatment with the sperm of someone else: someone, preferably, who has consented to the use of his sperm. If the HFEA had maintained its refusal to send Mr Blood's sperm to Belgium, this, in our view would not have been an infringement of such rights to medical treatment that Mrs Blood could reasonably be said to have. If it were in breach of a legal right which Mrs Blood and other people in similar situations have, then we suggest that the law or laws from which the right is derived should be reconsidered.

It might be said, by analogy, that Mrs Blood, like any one else so placed, has a right to remarry : however, she does not have, in the same sense of the term a 'right', a legal right to marry a particular person. People (including the desired spouses) and agencies might do things which have the effect of preventing Mrs Blood and others from marrying particular people without thereby infringing the legal rights of Mrs Blood and these people to marry.

If Mrs Blood had a legal right to the use of Mr Blood's sperm to impregnate herself in this particular case, as we have just described it, this right could have been exercised only by the commission of illegal acts. Even if she had such a right, perhaps it was against the public interest to uphold it.

One might want to raise the question of what counts as 'medical treatment'. Although medical procedures are sometimes required to fertilise some particular people, the question suggests itself: is fertility treatment medical treatment? Is medical treatment so constituted by its end or its means (or by some other thing or things)? Would sexual intercourse count as 'medical treatment' were it performed by medical practitioners and performed for the purposes of fertilising a 'patient'? Are, for instance, heart bypass surgical operations and cosmetic surgery equally 'medical treatment'? Perhaps they are: we are not begging the question.

Mrs Blood did not need to become pregnant. If she wanted to become pregnant, she did not need fertility treatment: she is not an infertile woman. She needed artificial insemination treatment only to become pregnant by her late husband. However much she wanted to do this, she did not need, however, to do so. Perhaps, of course, need has nothing intrinsically to do with medical treatment.

Posthumous Conception and Paternity

Perhaps the law concerning posthumous conception and paternity should be changed. On the other hand, perhaps there are good reasons against changing it. There are, undoubtedly, good reasons against changing it thoughtlessly. A dispassionate, relaxed and rational debate about the matter would be a good idea. The matter is not, despite what the *Herald* newspaper and Mrs Blood suggest, a trivial technicality.

If the law were changed in the suggested way, then there would be a particular and novel problem created about inheritance and about the settling of estates. This does not mean that the law should not be changed but it does mean that a lot of deliberation would be required before the change – were it to be made – could be made with justified confidence.

If the law were changed, how – if at all – would this affect the willingness of people to donate their sperm and other parts of their bodies? Were the law to be changed retrospectively, what effects might this have with regard to organ and related donation?

There is a *prima facie* case against retrospective legislation. Retrospective legislation of whatever sort can cause wariness of, and lack of confidence in, the law in general. It is a legal fiction that ignorance of the law is no excuse: morally, ignorance of the law is often a watertight excuse. This is one reason but by no means the only one why retrospective legislation is upsetting, unsettling and, in general, greatly to be discouraged. With retrospective legislation, it is as if, during a game, the referee, rather than upholding the rules of the game, were to apply the rules of some other game.

In the particular case concerning Mrs Blood, there might seem to be nothing to be lost and advantages to be gained by declaring that Stephen Blood is the legal father of Liam. However, soft as well as hard cases can make for bad laws [10].

Conclusion

If, to answer Scott's question, a case similar to that of Mr and Mrs Blood's were to recur, what should be done?

Suppose that, in the U.K., a married couple want and intend to have children. Suppose that one of them goes into a coma and that the remaining, conscious one requests the surgical removal of the other's sperm or ova. If consent has not been given to this procedure, then the doctors should not carry it out. Suppose that the procedure is carried out, sperm or ova are lodged with a licensed clinic and that the comatose person dies. Suppose that the remaining partner requests the use of the gametes with a view to become either the mother or the father of the dead partner's child. If written permission has not been given for this procedure, then the HFEA should refuse the request and seek to ensure the destruction of the gametes on the grounds that their very storage would be illegal in the absence of written consent. Perhaps there should be a prosecution of the guilty party.

The destruction of the gametes would be a suitable ending of the case. If, however, they were not destroyed and permission were requested by the widow or widower to have them sent abroad for use on the grounds that the widow or widower had a legal right under European Union Law to their use for medical treatment there, this request should be denied. It should be denied on the grounds that the denial is not an infringement of any legal rights to medical treatment which the widow or widower could reasonably be considered to have. That which one wants, no matter how profoundly, does not automatically become something to which one has a legal (or moral) right. After all, the widow or widower has no more legal right to the use of these particular gametes than has any other member of the European Union and that is to say: no legal right at all. If the widow or widower has a legal right to medical treatment in, for example, Belgium, then let her or him go there and receive it (or not receive it as the case may be). The actions and decisions of the HFEA that are here envisaged and suggested do not infringe such a right if there is one. The right – if it exists – is a right to a particular sort of treatment rather than treatment with particular gametes. What should happen additionally is that the relevant U.K. court and appeal court uphold this position.

*By Hugh V. McLachlan and J. Kim Swales, from *Human Reproduction and Genetic Ethics*, 2003, Vol.9, No. 1, pp. 7-12.

Bibliography

(1) Scott, A. (2002), 'Legal Responses to some of the New Developments in Reproductive Technologies, Part 2: The Case of Diane Blood', *Human Reproduction and Genetic Ethics,* Vol. 8, No. 1, p. 15.
(2) Scott, A. (2002), 'Legal Responses to some of the New Developments in Reproductive Technologies, Part 2 : The Case

of Diane Blood', *Human Reproduction and Genetic Ethics,* Vol. 8, No. 1, p. 11.

(3) Fergusson, P. (1997), 'Posthumous Conception: Blood and Gametes', *Scots Law Times,* Issue 8, February 28.

(4) See, for instance, *The Herald,* February 9, 2002.

(5) *The Herald,* February 9, 2002.

(6) *The Herald,* February 9, 2002.

(7) Warnock, M. (1984), *Report of the Committee of Inquiry into Human Fertilisation and Embryology.* Cmnd. 9314, para. 10.9.

(8) Warnock, M. (1984), *Report of the Committee of Inquiry into Human Fertilisation and Embryology.* Cmnd. 9314, para. 4.4.

(9) McHale, J. and Fox. M. with Murphy, J. (1997), *Health Care Law. Text and Materials,* Sweet and Maxwell, London, p. 941.

(10) See Brazier, M. (1997), 'Guest Editorial: Hard Cases Make Bad Laws?', *Journal of Medical Ethics,* Vol. 23, No. 6, pp. 341-343.

Chapter Twenty-four

Posthumous Insemination and Consent: A Reply to Mrs Blood*

Mrs Blood accuses us of giving an inaccurate account, in relation to the law, of the case pertaining to the use of her late husband's sperm [1] We reject this charge. We would counter by suggesting that Mrs Blood misrepresents our position by quoting and/or appearing to quote us in an unfair and misleading way. However, she also says that we were at fault in saying that the treatment used to procure sperm from Mr Blood would have irreparably damaged his testicles had he survived. We were not originating this claim but repeating what we believed to be an uncontested medical fact. We apologise for doing so. We are sorry for any distress that we thereby caused Mrs Blood and her family.

Mrs Blood says that: '... my main dispute with the facts of my case as portrayed by Dr. Hugh V. McLachlan and Prof. J Kim Swales is that of the Court of Appeal Judgment' [2]. She then goes on to say:

'On the subject of the court's ruling that I had a right to export the sperm under European Union Law, they say that: "the right – if it exists – is to a particular sort of treatment rather than treatment with particular gametes". The right does exist. That was the whole point of the judgment and my legal victory and the right established did facilitate treatment with the sperm of my late husband in particular[3].

This is a distortion of our views and of the nature and purpose of our article [4]. We were not disagreeing about what, as a matter of fact the Court of Appeal concluded. We were not denying that Mrs Blood was said by the Court of have a legal right to arrange for the export Mr Blood's sperm to Belgium. Our claims pertained to the soundness of the judgments and the wisdom of the laws about which the judgement was derived. We were not disputing what the courts mentioned here have ruled or will rule but what they should rule and should have ruled.

It was in the context of discussing, in the abstract, what should happen in an envisaged future case where a widow or widower in the UK claimed with reference to the European Union the legal right to become a mother or father rather than what did occur in an actual one that we wrote: 'The right – if it exists – is a right to a particular sort of treatment rather than treatment with particular gametes. What should happen additionally is that the relevant U.K. court and appeal court uphold this position' [5]. The section of our article in which this opinion of ours was made was introduced by the sentence: 'If, to answer Scott's question, a case similar to that of Mr and Mrs Blood's were to recur, what should be done [6]? We were offering an opinion rather than making a factually true or false claim when we when said the words that Mrs Blood quotes as being central to her charge against us of inaccuracy.

It was also in the context of discussing what should happen were a similar sort of case to occur that we said: 'Perhaps there should be a prosecution of the guilty party' [7]. We were not contemplating nor suggesting the prosecution of Mrs Blood, despite the impression her comment might create. Indeed, we had and have no criticism to make of her actions in relation to this case. We said that the treatment used to procure sperm from Mr Blood, who was in a coma at the time, was, technically, an assault since it was done without his consent, was not done to save or promote his own life or health and was not otherwise in his own best interests. Furthermore the use and even the storage of Mr Blood's sperm were contrary to the Human Fertilisation and Embryology Act of 1990 since he had not given his written consent. However, we did not suggest that Mrs Blood assaulted her husband. Mrs Blood calls our article a ferocious attack on her and her family. It was not an attack of any sort on her or them. We did not blame her for making the requests that she did concerning her husband and his sperm. We questioned, rather, the wisdom and legality acceding to them.

Central to our interest in and concern with the case of Mr and Mrs Blood is the nature and importance of consent – informed consent and, sometimes, written consent. Mr Blood did not give written consent to the use of his sperm and he did not give consent to the medical treatment applied to him when he was alive to obtain the sperm. Mrs Blood says: 'He could not consent in writing at the time his sperm was taken, as he was in a coma, but had previously expressed his wishes in the form of a conversation... and details were relayed to the doctors at the time they removed the sperm. This is contrary to the impression given by the article I take issue with that "the doctors did not even have Mr Blood's oral consent to the taking (let alone the use) of his gametes" [8].'

We do not doubt for a moment Mrs Blood's veracity. That she truly and truthfully expressed what her husband said to her is not in dispute. The relevance of such a reported conversation is what is at issue. We maintain that it should not be thought of as tantamount to consent on the part of Mr Blood. If he had been, in the relevant context, asked to give consent, he might well (as Mrs Blood's evidence suggests) have done so. But he was not so asked and he did not give consent.

Wanting to do something is not the same as consenting to do so; wanting something to happen is not the same as consenting to its being done. For instance, there would be no need to bother with having general elections and there could be recourse instead to opinion polls if wanting something were the same as consenting to it. Even saying that one wants something to be done is not necessarily the same as consenting to it: the context is crucial. A bride might truly report at the alter that her fiancé said that he wanted to marry her and also said that he would, if and when the relevant time came, consent to do so. This is not tantamount to consent on the part of the groom. It does not constitute the saying by him in an appropriate place at the appropriate time: 'I do'.

Wanting to have sex with a particular person is not the same as authorising that person to have sexual congress by the self conscious, voluntary expression of informed consent. Even saying to a person that one wants at some future time to have sex with him does not in itself constitute consent to future instances of sexual intercourse. Apart from any thing else – and these are not the only considerations – people can change their minds; people can be mistaken about their own future desires and intentions; and people can lie. It was in this context that we said – and would continue to say – that the invasive treatment used to obtain sperm from the comatose Mr Blood was akin to rape. It was not rape although it was an assault.

Consent in general is important and it is of particular importance in relation to the treatment by others of our bodies and of our corporal issues and tissues. If the significance of the notion of consent were in any way diminished and diluted by the decisions made in the case of Mr and Mrs Blood then this would indeed be troubling. Recently, there was a proposal made that school-children should be tested in order to ascertain whether or not they have been taking drugs. It was apparent that a requirement for consent for this treatment from the children themselves and/or from their parents was, to say the least, not pivotal to the thinking of the politicians involved. Vigilance concerning consent is of perennial importance.

*By Hugh V. McLachlan and J. Kim Swales.

References

(1) See Blood, D. (2004), 'To Correct the record: The Continuing, troubling, inaccurate account of my case', *Human Reproduction and Genetic Ethics*, Vol. 10, No. 1, pp. 2-4.

(2) Ibid. p. 2.

(3) Ibid. p. 2.

(4) See McLachlan, H.V. and Swales, J.K., (2003), 'Posthumous Insemination and Consent: The Continuing, Troubling Case of Mr and Mrs Blood', *Human Reproduction and Genetic Ethics*, Vol. 9, No. 1, pp. 7-12.

(5) Ibid. p.11.

(6) Ibid. p. 11.

(7) Ibid. p. 11.

(8) Blood, D. (2004), 'To Correct the record: The Continuing, troubling, inaccurate account of my case', *Human Reproduction and Genetic Ethics*, Vol. 10, No. 1, p. 2.

Bibliography

Acton, H.B.(1970) *Kant's Moral Philosophy*, Macmillan, London.

Advisers to the President of the European Commission on the Ethical Implications of Biotechnology (1997) 'Ethical Aspects of Cloning Techniques', *Journal of Medical Ethics*, Vol. 23, No. 6, pp. 349-352

Aigen, Betsey P.(1996) 'Motivations of Surrogate Mothers: Parenthood, Altruism and Self-Actualization', TASC@surrogacy.com

Anderson, E.(1993) *Value in Ethics and Economics,* Harvard University Press: The MIT Press, Cambridge, MA.

Andersson, J.O.(1995) 'Real Freedom, Democratic Community and Sustainable Development as Fundamental Values in Economic Enquiry' in *Economic Value and Ways of Life,* edited by R. Eriksson and M. Jantii, Avebury, Aldershot.

Arneson, R.(1992) Commodification and Commercial Surrogacy. *Philosophy and Public Affairs* 21, pp. 132-164.

Barry B. (1995) *Justice as Impartiality,* Vol II of *A Treatise on Social Justice.* Clarendon Press, Oxford.

Beyleverd D. and Brownsword R.(1998) 'Human Dignity, Human Rights and Human Genes', *The Modern Law Review*, 1998, Vol. 61.

Blood, D. (2004) 'To Correct the record: The Continuing, troubling, inaccurate account of my case', *Human Reproduction and Genetic Ethics*, Vol. 10, No. 1, pp. 2-4.

Brazier, M.(1992) *Medicine, Patients and the Law*, Penguin Books.

Brazier, M. (1997) 'Hard Cases Make Bad Law' *Journal of Medical Ethics Vol.* 23, pp. 341-343.

Brazier, M., Campbell, A. and Golombok, S.(1998) *Surrogacy: Review for Health Ministers of Current Arrangements for Payments and Regulations;* Report of the Review Team, Cm 4068.

Broadie, Alexander (2000) *Why Scottish Philosophy Matters*, The Saltire Society, Edinburgh.

Bruce, Donald 2001, 'Human Embryonic Cloning', *Human Reproduction and Genetic Ethics*, Vol. 7, No. 1, pp. 3-7.

Bruce, Donald 2002, 'Running on the Spot: The ethics of the new technologies', *Life and Work*, April, pp. 19-21.

Bruce, D. and Bruce. A (eds), 1998, *Engineering Genesis*, Earthscan, London.

Buchanan, A., Brock D., Daniels N. and Wikler D. (2000) *From Chance to Choice: Genetics and Justice*, Cambridge University Press, Cambridge.

Burley, J. (ed.), (1999) *The Genetic Revolution and Human Rights*, Oxford University Press, Oxford.

Burley, J and Harris, J, (eds.), (2002) *A Companion to Genetic Ethics,* Blackwell, Maiden, Mass.

Campbell, A.V.(2000) 'Surrogacy, Rights and Duties: A Partial Commentary', *Health Care Analysis,* 8, pp. 35-40.

Campbell, T. *et al.* (eds), 1986, *Human Rights: From Rhetoric to Reality*, Oxford, Blackwell.

Caulfield, T. (2003) 'Human Cloning Laws, Human Dignity and the Poverty of the Policy Making Dialogue' *BMC Medical Ethics*, Vol. 4, No. 3.

Church of Scotland (1996) *Pre-conceived Ideas: A Christian Perspective of IVF and Embryology*, St. Andrews Press, Edinburgh.

Culyer, A.J.(2001)'Equity — some theory and its policy implications', *Journal of Medical Ethics* Vol. **27**, pp. 275–83.

Daar, A.S.(1998)'Paid Organ Donation – The Grey Basket Concept', *Journal of Medical Ethics* 24, pp. 365-368.

Dickens, C. (1992) *The old curiosity shop,* Collins, London and Glasgow.

Dworkin, R.(2002) *Sovereign virtue: The theory and practice of equality*, Harvard University Press, London.

Fergusson, P. (1997) 'Posthumous Conception: Blood and Gametes', *Scots Law Times*, Issue 8, February 28.

Fox, Marie (2000) 'Pre-persons, Commodities or Cyborgs? The Legal Construction and Representation of the Embryo', *Health Care Analysis*, Vol. 8, pp. 171-181.

Freeden, M. (1991) *Rights*, Milton Keynes, Open University.

Freeman, M. (1989) 'Is Surrogacy Exploitative?' in *Legal Issues in Human Reproduction,* Sheila McLean, (editor), Aldershot, Gower.

Galbraith, Mhairi, McLachlan, Hugh V. and Swales, J.Kim (2005) 'Commercial Surrogacy Agencies: A Transactions Costs Approach,' (with M. Galbraith and J.K. Swales), *Health Care Analysis*, Vol.13, No.1.

Gogarty, B. (2003) 'What exactly is an exact copy? And why it matters when trying to ban reproductive cloning in Australia', *Journal of Medical Ethics*, vol. 29, pp. 84-89.

Gostin, L. (1988) 'A Civil Liberties Analysis of Surrogacy Arrangements', *Law, Medicine and Health Care,* Vol. 16, pp. 7-17.

Gostin, L. (2001) 'Surrogacy From the Perspectives of Economic and Civil Liberties', *The Journal of Contemporary Health Law and Policy,* Vol. 17, pp. 429-431.

Green, R.M.(2001) *The Human Embryo Research Debates: Bioethics in the Vortex of Controversy*, Oxford University Press.

Hare, R. M.(1975)'Abortion and the Golden Rule', *Philosophy and Public Affairs*, Vol. 4.

Harris, John (1997) '"Goodbye Dolly?" The Ethics of Human Cloning', *Journal of Medical Ethics*, Vol. 23, No. 6, pp. 353360.

Harris, John (1998) *Clones, Genes and Immortality: Ethics and the Genetic Revolution*, Oxford University Press, Oxford.
Harris, John (1999) 'Clones, Genes and Human Rights' in J Burley, editor, *The Genetic Revolution and Human Rights*, Oxford, Oxford University Press, pp. 61-94.
Harris, John (2000) 'The Welfare of the Child', *Health Care Analysis* 8, pp. 27-34.
Harris, John (2004) 'Before Birth – After Death', *Journal of Medical Ethics*. No. 30, p. 425.
Hindess, Barry (1982) 'Power, Interests and the Outcome of Struggles', *Sociology*, Vol. 16, No. 4.
Hohfeld, W.N. (1978) *Fundamental Legal Conceptions as Applied to Judicial Reasoning*, Greenwood Press, Westport.
Keown, J. (1997) 'The Gift of Blood in Europe: An Ethical Defence of EC Directive 89/581', *Journal of Medical Ethics*, Vol. 23.
Keown, J. (1998)'A Reply to McLachlan' *Journal of Medical Ethics*, Vol. 24.
King, David (2003), 'Just How Complex is Genetics Really?', *Human Reproduction and Genetic Ethics*, Vol. 9, No. 1, pp. 13-15.
Kornegay, R.J. (1990) Is Commercial Surrogacy Baby Selling? *Journal of Applied Philosophy* 7, pp. 45-50.
Kymlicka, Will (1991) 'Re-thinking the Family: Review of Okin's Justice, Gender and the Family', *Philosophy and Public Affairs,* Vol. 20, pp. 77-97.
Land, W. and Dossetor, J.B. (eds.) (1991) *Organ Replacement Therapy: Ethics, Justice and Commerce,* Springer-Verlag, Berlin.
Lederberg, Joshua (2003), 'Learning from our complex relationship with bugs', *The Herald*, April 26, p. 15.
Le Grand, J. (1991) *Equity and Choice: An Essay in Economics and Applied Philosophy,* Harper Collins Academic, London and New York.
Levine, David P. (1997) *Self-Seeking and the Pursuit of Justice*, Ashgate, Aldershot.
McHale, J. and Fox M. with Murhpy, J. (1991) *Health Care Law: Text and Materials*, London, Sweet and Maxwell.
McLachlan, Hugh V. (1973) 'The Right to Work', *Contemporary Review*, June, pp. 307-311.
McLachlan, Hugh V. (1977) 'Must We Accept Either the Conservative or the Liberal View on Abortion?' *Analysis* 37, pp. 197-204.
McLachlan, Hugh V. (1979) 'The Is/Ought Question: A Needless Controversy', *Journal of the British Society for Phenomenology*, Vol. 10, No. 2, pp. 134-137.
McLachlan, Hugh V. (1981) 'Wittgenstein, Family Resemblances and the Theory of Classification', *International Journal of Sociology and Social Policy* 1(1), pp. 1-16.

McLachlan, Hugh V. (1983) Townsend and the Concept of "Poverty"', *Social Policy and Administration,* Vol. 17, No. 2, pp. 97-105.
McLachlan, Hugh V.(1985), 'In Defence of Surrogate Motherhood', *Contemporary Review,* January.
McLachlan, Hugh V. (1986) 'Concepts of Poverty and Deprivation', *Journal of Social Policy,* Vol. 15, No. 4, pp. 499-501.
McLachlan, Hugh V.(1993) 'Warnock and Research on Human Embryos: A Case for a Re-Appraisal of the Fertilisation and Embryology Act (1990)', *International Journal of Sociology and Social Policy* 13, pp. 110-119.
McLachlan, Hugh V. (1994), 'Freedom and the Market: A Defence of "Socialist" Intervention', *The Philosopher*, Autumn.
McLachlan, Hugh V.(1995)'On Producing Embryos for Research', *The Philosopher,* 21, pp. 2-11.
McLachlan, Hugh V. (1995) 'No Two Sets Exactly the Same? Applying Philosophy to the Theory of Fingerprints', *The Philosopher*, Vol. 83, No. 2, pp. 12-18.
McLachlan, Hugh V. (1995) 'Smokers, Virgins, Equity and Health Care Costs' *Journal of Medical Ethics* Vol. 21, pp. 209-213.
McLachlan, Hugh V. (1997) 'Defending Commercial Surrogate Motherhood Against Van Nierkerk and Van Zyl', *Journal of Medical Ethics* 23, pp. 344-348.
McLachlan, Hugh V. (1997) 'Bodies, Rights and Abortion', *Journal of Medical Ethics*, Vol. 23, No. 3, pp. 176-180.
McLachlan, Hugh V. (1997) 'Defending Commercial Surrogate Motherhood Against Van Niekerk and Van Zyl', *Journal of Medical Ethics* Vol. 23, pp. 344-348.
McLachlan, Hugh V. (1998) 'The Un-Paid Donation of Blood and Altruism: A Comment on Keown', *Journal of Medical Ethics,* Vol. 24, 252-254.
McLachlan, Hugh V. (1998) 'Justice, Rights and Health Care: A Discussion of the Report of the Commission on Social Justice, *International Journal of Sociology and Social Policy* Vol. 18 no. 11/12.
McLachlan, Hugh V.(1999) 'Altruism, Blood Donation and Public Policy: A Reply to Keown', *Journal of Medical Ethics,* Vol. 25, No.6.
McLachlan, Hugh V.(2000) 'Scotland, social justice, health and inequality' in Nottingham C, ed. *The NHS in Scotland: the legacy of the past and the prospect of the future*, Ashgate, Aldershot.
McLachlan, Hugh V.(2005)'Ignore The Boys from Brazil – say "Yes" to human cloning' *The Scotsman*, 5th November.
McLachlan, Hugh V. (2005) 'Poor reasons for making human cloning illegal' *The Scotsman*, 26 Nov.

McLachlan Hugh V. (2004) 'Human Embryos, Clones and Public Policy: A Critique of the Church of Scotland's Views' *Scottish Affairs*, No. 46, pp. 110-130.
McLachlan Hugh V. (2005) *Social Justice, Human Rights and Public Policy* Glasgow, Humming Earth, Glasgow.
McLachlan, Hugh V. and Swales, J.K. (1993), 'Sexual Bias and the Law: The Case of Pre-Industrial Scotland', *International Journal of Sociology and Social Policy*, Vol. 14, No. 9.
McLachlan, Hugh V. and Swales, J.Kim. (1997), 'Provider of Service Worthy of Payment', *The Scotsman*, 12th June, p. 6.
McLachlan, Hugh V. and Swales, J.Kim (1998) 'Commercial Surrogate Motherhood' *Contemporary Review*, pp. 113-117.
McLachlan, Hugh V and Swales, J. Kim (1998) The Methodology Rather than the Rhetoric of Economics: McCloskey on Popper and Hume', *Journal of Interdisciplinary Economics 9* (2), pp. 125-143.
McLachlan, Hugh V. and Swales, J.Kim (1999) 'A Drunk Driver, A Sober Pedestrian and the Allocation of Tragically Scarce and Indivisible Emergency Hospital Treatment', *Health Care Analysis* 7(1), pp. 5-21.
McLachlan, Hugh V. and Swales, J.Kim (2000)'Babies, Child Bearers and Commodification: Anderson, Brazier *et al.* and the Political Economy of Commercial Surrogate Motherhood', Health Care Analysis, 8 (1), pp. 1-18.
McLachlan, Hugh V. and Swales, J.Kim (2000)'Scotland, the Church and Surrogate Motherhood', Scottish Affairs, Summer, 32.
McLachlan, Hugh V. and Swales, J.Kim (2003) 'Posthumous Insemination and Consent: The Continuing, Troubling Case of Mr and Mrs Blood', *Human Reproduction and Genetic Ethics*, Vol. 9, No. 1, pp. 7-12.
McLean, Sheila (ed.) (1989) *Legal Issues in Human Reproduction,* Aldershot, Gower.
Malby, S.(2002) 'Human Dignity and Human Reproductive Cloning' *Health and Human Rights,* Vol. 6, pp. 103-135.
Maxwell-Stuart, P.G., 2001, *Satan's Conspiracy: Magic and Witchcraft in Sixteenth-Century Scotland,* Tuckwell Press, East Linton.
Mill, J.S. (1966) 'On Liberty', in M. Warnock (Ed.), *Utilitarianism,* Collins, London.
Munzer, S.R.(1990), *A Theory of Property*, Cambridge University Press, Cambridge.
Nottingham C. (ed.)(2000) *The NHS in Scotland: the legacy of the past and the prospect of the future*, Ashgate, Aldershot.
O'Neill O.(2002) *Autonomy and Trust in Bioethics,*: Cambridge University Press, Cambridge.
Pattison S. (2002) 'Reproductive Cloning: Can Cloning Harm the Clone?', *Medical Law Review*, 10 pp. 295-307.

Raphael D.D.(1971) *Problems of political philosophy*, Macmillan, London.

Rawls J. (1971) *A Theory of Justice*, Harvard University Press, Cambridge.

Resnik, D. (1998) 'The Commodification of Human Reproductive Materials', *Journal of Medical Ethics* 24, pp. 388-393.

Ridley, M. (2003) *Nature Via Nurture: Genes, Experience and What Makes Us Human*, Fourth Estate, London.

Robertson, John (1983) *Surrogate Mothers: Not so Novel after All*, Hastings Centre Report, October, pp. 28-34.

Robertson J. (1994) 'The Question of Human Cloning', *Hastings Center Report*, 24, pp. 6-14.

Robertson J. (1998) 'Liberty, Identity and Human Cloning', *Texas Law Review*, 76, pp. 1371-1456.

Rovane C. (2002) 'Genetics and Personal Identity' in *A Companion to Genetic Ethics,* edited by J. Burley and J. Harris, Blackwell, Maiden, Mass., pp. 245-252.

Savulescu J. (2002) 'Is there a "right not to be born"?: Reproductive decision making, options and the right to information', *Journal of Medical Ethics*, Vol.28, pp. 65-67.

Schachter, O. (1983) 'Human Dignity as a Normative Concept' *American Journal of International Law*, 77, pp. 848-854.

Scott, A. (2002), 'Legal Responses to some of the New Developments in Reproductive Technologies, Part 2: The Case of Diane Blood', *Human Reproduction and Genetic Ethics*, Vol. 8, No. 1.

Scruton, Roger (1982) *A Dictionary of Political Thought*, Pan Books.

Shalev, C. (2002) 'Human Cloning and Human Rights: A Commentary', *Health and Human Rights*, 6 pp. 137-151.

Shaver, S.(1993/94)'Body rights, social rights and the liberal welfare state', *Critical Social Policy* 39 pp. 70.

Singer, Peter and Wells, Deane (1985), *Making Babies: The New Science and Ethics of Contraception,* New York, Charles Scribner's Sons.

Smith, A. (1976) *The Theory of Moral Sentiments,* Edited by D.D. Raphael and A.Macfie, Clarendon Press, Oxford.

Smith, Ken (1998), 'Surrogacy for cash defended', *The Herald*, 9th, April, p. 10

Smith V.R. and Bopp A. E. (1999) 'Smokers and taxes', *Journal of Medical Ethics,* 1999, Vol. 25, p.419.

Stewart, Graeme (1998) 'Commercial surrogacy not immoral, say academics', *The Scotsman*, 8th April, p. 10.

Thomson, J.J. (1972) 'A Defense of Abortion', *Philosophy and Public Affairs*, Vol. 2.

Thornton, J.(1999) *Should Health Screening be Private?,* The I.E.A. Health and Welfare Unit, Choice in Welfare No. 48.

Tobin J. (1970) 'On limiting the domain of inequality' *Journal of Law and Economics*, Vol. 5, pp. 263–78.
Tong, R. (1997) *Feminist Approaches to Bioethics*, Westview Press, Oxford.
Tooley, M. (1972) 'Abortion and Infanticide', *Philosophy and Public Affairs*, Vol. 2.
Townsend, Peter (1984) 'A Rejoinder on Poverty', *Social Policy and Administration*, Vol. 18, No. 2, pp. 165-167.
van Niekerk, A. and van Zyl, L. (1995a) 'Commercial Surrogacy and the Commodification of Children: An Ethical Perspective', *Medicine and Law* 14, pp. 163-170.
van Niekerk, A. and van Zyl, L. (1995b) 'The Ethics of Surrogacy: Women's Reproductive Labour' *Journal of Medical Ethics* 21, pp. 345-349.
Veit-Wilson, John (1986) 'Paradigms of Poverty: A Rehabilitation of B.S. Rowntree', *Journal of Social Policy*, Vol. 5, No. 1, pp. 69-99.
Waldron J. (1988) *The right to private property*, Clarendon Press, Oxford.
Warnock, M. (1984) *Report of the Committee of Inquiry into Human Fertilisation and Embryology*, Cmnd. 9314.
Warnock, M. (1985) A *Question of Life: The Warnock Report on Human Fertilisation and Embryology*, Blackwell, Oxford.
Werner, R. (1976) 'Hare on Abortion', *Analysis* Vol. 36, No. 4.
Werthheimer, A. 1996) *Exploitation*, Princeton University Press, Princeton.
Wright T.G. (2000) 'Second Thoughts: How Human Cloning Can Promote Human Dignity', *Valparaiso University Law Review*, 35, pp. 1-35.

Index

Lightning Source UK Ltd.
Milton Keynes UK
28 November 2009

146873UK00001B/44/A

9 781846 220111